Laparoscopy in Urology

Dedicated to John (*mentor meus*)

Laparoscopy in Urology

MALCOLM J. COPTCOAT
ChM FRCS (Urol)
Consultant Urologist and Director of Surgery
King's College Hospital, London

AND

ADRIAN D. JOYCE
MS FRCS (Urol)
Consultant Urologist
Leeds General Infirmary

IN TWO PARTS
PART 1

The views expressed in this book are not necessarily those of ZENECA Pharma

OXFORD
BLACKWELL SCIENTIFIC PUBLICATIONS
LONDON EDINBURGH BOSTON
MELBOURNE PARIS BERLIN VIENNA

Editorial Offices:
Osney Mead, Oxford OX2 0EL
25 John Street, London WC1N 2BL
23 Ainslie Place, Edinburgh EH3 6AJ
238 Main Street, Cambridge
Massachusetts 02142, USA
54 University Street, Carlton
Victoria 3053, Australia

Other Editorial Offices:
Librairie Arnette SA
2, rue Casimir-Delavigne
75006 Paris
France

Blackwell Wissenschafts-Verlag GmbH
Düsseldorfer Str. 38
D-10707 Berlin
Germany

Blackwell MZV
Feldgasse 13
A-1238 Wien
Austria

First published 1993

Set by DSM, Oxford
Printed and bound in Great Britain
at the the University Press, Cambridge

DISTRIBUTORS

Marston Book Services Ltd
PO Box 87
Oxford OX2 0DT
(*Orders*: Tel: 0865 791155
Fax: 0865 791927
Telex: 837515)

USA
Blackwell Scientific Publications, Inc.
238 Main Street
Cambridge, MA 02142
(*Orders*: Tel: 800 759-6102
617 876-7000)

Canada
Times Mirror Professional Publishing, Ltd
130 Flaska Drive
Markham, Ontario L6G 1B8
(*Orders*: Tel. 800 268-4178
416 470-6739)

Australia
Blackwell Scientific Publications Pty Ltd
54 University Street
Carlton, Victoria 3053
(*Orders*: Tel: 03 347-5552)

A catalogue record for this title is available from the British Library and the Library of Congress

ISBN 0-632-03664-8

Contents

List of Contributors

MALCOLM J. COPTCOAT ChM FRCS (Urol)
Consultant Urologist and Director of Surgery, King's College Hospital, Denmark Hill, London SE5 9RS, England

CHRISTOPHER G. EDEN MB BS FRCS
Wickham Fellow and Honorary Urological Registrar, King's College Hospital, Denmark Hill, London SE5 9RS, England

DAVID GREEN FRC Anaes
Consultant Anaesthetist, King's College Hospital, Denmark Hill, London SE5 9RS, England

ADRIAN D. JOYCE MS FRCS (Urol)
Consultant Urologist, Leeds General Infirmary, Great George Street, Leeds LS1 3EX, England

MARCIN MATUSZEWSKI MD
Resident in Urology and Visiting Fellow to King's College Hospital, Medical Academy, Kieturakisa 1, Gdansk, Poland

ANGUS MITCHELL FRC Anaes
Senior Anaesthetic Registrar, King's College Hospital, Denmark Hill, London SE5 9RS, England

Preface

Surgical practice is undergoing a revolution. Minimally invasive techniques are rapidly replacing traditional open surgical procedures. The epitome of the change is to be found in laparoscopy.

In 1990, laparoscopy in urology was confined to diagnosis of the intra-abdominal testicle. Many of us had witnessed the complex operative gynaecological laparoscopy of Professor Kurt Semm but were frustrated by a lack of the instrumentation needed in urology. However, an explosion in the use of laparoscopic cholecystectomy has now not only changed general surgery but led to the innovative developments in equipment that allow us to perform complex laparoscopic procedures in urology.

Laparoscopy is a team effort, and the establishment of a laparoscopic centre of excellence in King's College Hospital has been possible only through the support and skills of my surgical and nursing colleagues. Innovations in surgery in this decade may spring from an individual but are clarified and modified very quickly by the wider international team. I am especially indebted to Ralph Clayman, Howard Winfield, Lou Kavoussi and many others who have made unselfish and forthcoming contributions to our pooled practical knowledge of laparoscopy in urology.

Acknowledgements

I am indebted to my Personal Assistant, Susan Horrell, for her invaluable assistance in preparing this book. Chris Eden and I took the photographs.

M.J.C.

1: Introduction

M.J. COPTCOAT AND A.D. JOYCE

Lord Lister's portrait hangs in the consultants' room at King's College Hospital, London. His pioneering work with aseptic techniques and his introduction of general anaesthesia to British surgery have made him one of the pillars of surgical wisdom in Great Britain. His solemn features give no hint to the exciting frontiers that his work opened up for surgeons who followed him. Just over 100 years ago he is quoted as saying 'These are exciting times to be a surgeon.' There is obviously a double peak to this excitement with the explosion of endoscopic and, in particular, laparoscopic surgery.

Endoscopic surgery is rapidly becoming a popular alternative to traditional operative open procedures for a variety of diseases. Laparoscopic biliary tract surgery, laparoscopic appendicectomy, laparoscopic gynaecological procedures, laparoscopic urological procedures, the thoracoscopic treatment of pneumothorax and persistent pleural effusions as well as arthroscopic examination and treatment of joint spaces have all become accepted endoscopic procedures. If conducted safely, endoscopic surgery offers savings in total health care as a result of short hospital stays and a more rapid return to normal activities. These are factors that are appealing to commercial health-care providers and the public themselves. There is now an increased public awareness that endoscopic surgery is associated with less pain and less cosmetic disfigurement. This is exemplified by the recent overwhelming introduction of laparoscopic cholecystectomy, which had attracted only minor curiosity when it was first performed in 1987. The exponential acceptance of this procedure has been stimulated by patient demands.

Many of us may not wish to learn new procedures when we have been in practice for a number of years but more than ever before our personal preference for a particular procedure is going to be overhauled by current health education and patients' new expectations.

There is a disadvantage for state health care providers such as the National Health Service with the advent of endoscopic surgery. The capital outlay costs and minimal disposable costs of this type of surgery can probably be written into future budget plans. But the impact on theatre time and expertise will cause large repercussions in the way we structure our current surgical practice. Many of these endoscopic procedures take up to twice as long as their open counterparts. The ultimate advantages are not in question but at present there is not the operating time, theatre personnel or surgical expertise available to introduce this revolution suddenly. These are important

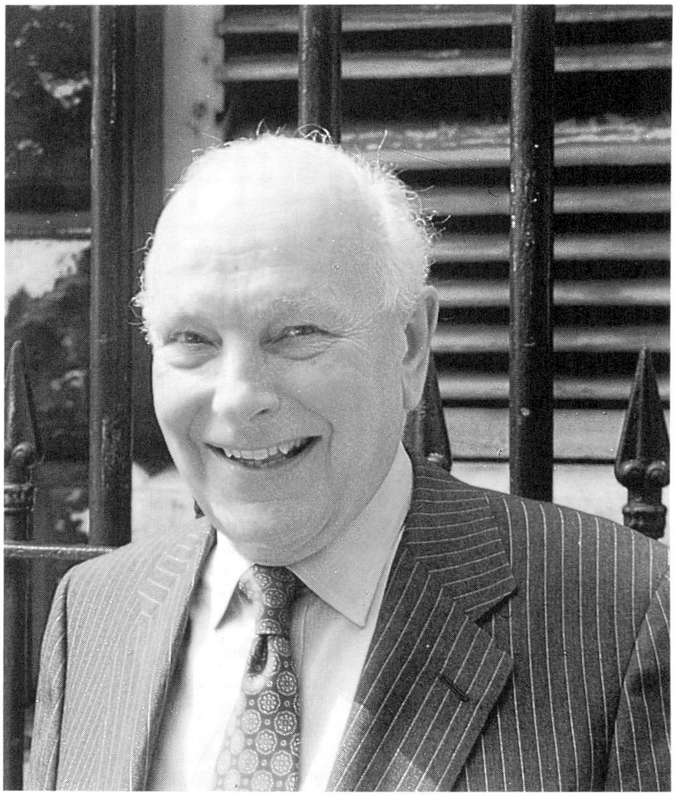

Fig. 1.1 Mr John Wickham, London, England: endoscopic pioneer and founder of the Minimally Invasive Therapy Society.

matters that must be addressed in the way we plan our departments and train our surgeons in the future. These horizons have been anticipated by only a few and no one stands out more than John Wickham (Fig. 1.1). Any difficulties that we might have in introducing these procedures to our hospitals can be blamed partly upon our lack of trust in this man's visionary thinking in the past. The formation of the Minimally Invasive Therapy Society and its close association with both industry and health-care economists will go a long way towards bringing these changes about.

Laparoscopy is transforming general surgery and general surgeons. The same revolution is going to occur in urology, and for once we have sat on our high-technology, minimally invasive laurels for a little too long.

Laparoscopy has previously been regarded as an interesting clinical diagnostic tool with very few applications. It has been well documented that laparoscopy could be helpful in localizing the impalpable undescended testicle when both ultrasound and computerized tomography (CT) have failed to help. But the numbers of these cases that an individual urologist sees are small and so the technique of laparoscopy has been left very much in the background. Laparoscopy need not be merely diagnostic. Here is a list of the operative laparoscopic procedures currently being performed in the urology department of King's College Hospital:

Laparoscopic abdominal orchidectomy
Laparoscopic abdominal orchidopexy (first stage)
Laparoscopic varicocelectomy
Laparoscopic inguinal herniorrhaphy
Laparoscopic appendicectomy
Laparoscopic pelvic lymphadenectomy
Laparoscopic para-aortic lymphadenectomy
Laparoscopic retroperitoneal surgery
- (a) Ureterolysis
- (b) Ureterolithotomy
- (c) Deroofing renal cyst
- (d) Nephrectomy
- (e) Pyeloplasty

Laparoscopic transperitoneal nephrectomy
- (a) Simple
- (b) Radical
- (c) Nephroureterectomy

Laparoscopic colposuspension
Laparoscopic bladder transsection
Laparoscopic ileal conduit diversion
Laparoscopic partial cystectomy
Laparoscopic lymphocele drainage

Many urologists may consider that whilst it might be feasible to carry out all of these procedures using a laparoscope, it will not be without a great deal of operative time and technology overlay. This perception is not justified.

One must return to the patient-priority concept of minimally invasive therapy (Wickham 1987), and that is to achieve the ideal operative result with minimal trauma and a rapid return to normal activities for the patient. This is witnessed in King's College Hospital when a postoperative laparoscopic nephrectomy case requires only oral analgesics, is able to tolerate an oral diet on the first operative day and goes home on the second postoperative day.

The above list of laparoscopic procedures is just a snapshot in the evolution of minimally invasive surgery, however. There have been three evolutionary steps so far. First, diagnosis; second, minor surgical techniques such as biopsy, clipping, cutting and, third, removal of large tissue volumes, such as a nephrectomy or splenectomy. The currently developing fourth step is that of laparoscopic reconstruction. Reconstruction, or rather the specific technique of tissue anastomosis, requires the re-evaluation of alternative technology such as glues, laser welding and absorbable stapling devices, because laparoscopic suturing is not just difficult to master but often inappropriate when working in a confined space. In a solution to this problem, we begin to see the divergence of laparoscopy from a method of merely copying open procedures. This will blossom when surgeons can rationalize the advantages that laparoscopy brings. Although a reduction in the trauma of access brings obvious advantages, there comes a point when the complexity of the intra-abdominal procedure produces greater potential morbidity. Thus, the internal part of our laparoscopic procedures must be more refined. Until this happens, the rationale for carrying out a laparoscopic radical cystectomy or prostatectomy will be based on feasibility for the surgeon and not decreased morbidity for the patient. The laparoscope is an internal operating microscope, and the dissection and manipulation should be precise. Our instrumentation does not yet always allow that, but it will come and with it the fifth evolutionary step of laparoscopy.

This book will undoubtedly age very rapidly. But during its short life span, we hope that it will serve as a practical guide to urologists wishing to take on operative laparoscopy. None of these procedures will by themselves be performed very frequently in a department but the increasing spectrum will allow experience to be gained and applied for any of them.

Reference

Wickham J.E.A. (1987) The 'new surgery'. *British Medical Journal*, **295**, 1581–2.

2: History of Laparoscopy

M.J. COPTCOAT AND M. MATUSZEWSKI

Laparoscopy is very much a development of the twentieth century. Kelling (1901) described a case report of inspection of the abdominal cavity of a dog using a Nitze cystoscope introduced through a small stab wound. The same author then described his use of this laparoscopic technique in man in 1923. Ott (1901) in Petrograd (now St Petersburg) described an alternative method for inspection of the abdominal contents by making a small incision and looking inside with a head mirror and indirect illumination. Ott called this technique 'ventroscopy'.

The father of what we now regard as laparoscopy, and indeed the first to use the term 'laparoscopy', was Jacobeus in Stockholm. In fact, 'laparo-' is literally translated from the Greek as 'flank', a combining form denoting a relationship to the loin or flank and sometimes used loosely in reference to the abdomen. This would not be the only instance when the most popular name has quite rightly its origin in a pioneer's technique rather than from a true etymological source. Jacobeus (1910) reported the use of a cystoscope for examination of both the peritoneal and pleural cavities. His instrument was inserted through a sheath trocar system. Both water and air were used for distention of the cavity, but the indication for the majority of his early patients was that of ascites when a concomitant paracentesis could be performed.

Little thought had been given at this time to the artificial introduction of air or water to increase the peritoneal cavity's dimensions. Bernheim (1911) from the Johns Hopkins Hospital in Baltimore called his technique of abdominal inspection 'organoscopy'. He utilized a proctoscope and was the first to state that the presence of ascites was not necessary. He used air for insufflation. He described two cases. One was referred by another famous surgeon, Halstead, with a pancreatic tumour. The organoscopy was carried out to look for metastases. None were identified, and in the true spirit of validation, they then proceeded to an open exploration to confirm the findings. They had been correct. A second case was described of a patient who presented with an acute abdomen for whom a provisional diagnosis of a gastric ulcer had been made. Acute appendicitis was identified during organoscopy and the patient subsequently underwent a successful appendicectomy, albeit by open incision. It is a little embarrassing to realize that the use of abdominal endoscopic inspection for the acute abdomen had been described in 1911 and we still find that many surgeons have not realized its potential in 1993 in this clinical situation.

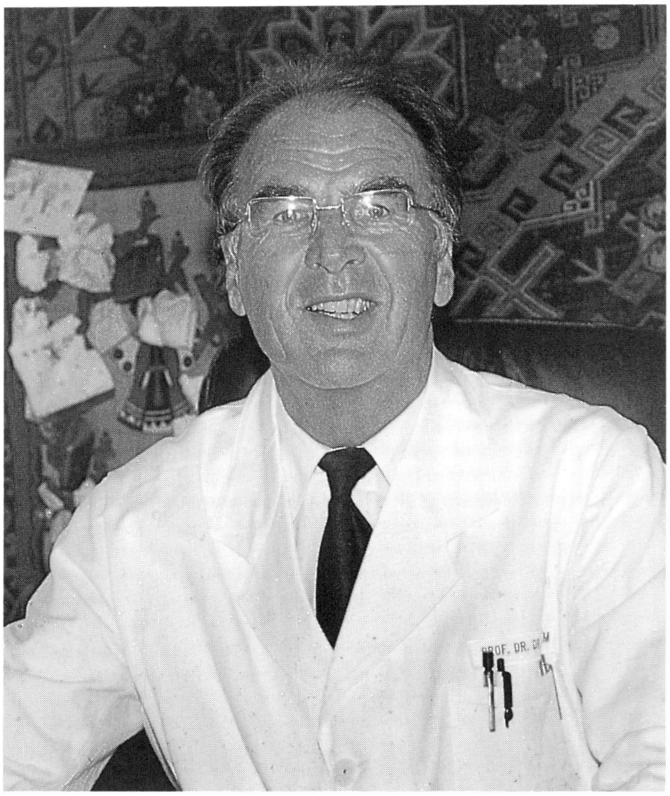

Fig. 2.1 Professor Kurt Semm, Kiel, Germany. The pioneer of operative laparoscopy in gynaecology. He also performed the first laparoscopic appendicectomy.

Nordentöft (1912) was the first to introduce a sharp-pointed trocar to ease the introduction of the sheath. At the same time, he advocated the use of the head-down or Trendelenberg position to make the insertion of the trocar and cannula safer.

Stolkind (1919) popularized the use of the laparoscope and made several innovative steps. He was the first to introduce the use of a smaller sharp cannula into the abdomen, through which air could be insufflated. This was then followed by the larger sharp-pointed trocar and cannula that would take the telescope. Zollikofer (1925) introduced the concept of carbon dioxide for insufflation, remarking that it was much safer than air, but not really going into great details as to why at this stage. With laparoscopy established as a safe diagnostic procedure, and with the instrumentation and technique accepted by most physicians and surgeons, we turn to Fervers (1933), who was the first to carry out some form of operative procedure. He described the technique of adhesiolysis. For this, he required the introduction of a second port for the insertion of scissors.

A very interesting contribution was made by Ruddock (1937) who reported on a series of 200 patients. He began the argument that has been taken up more recently regarding the economics of laparoscopy. He showed quite clearly that the decreased morbidity in his patients who were saved from open surgery easily outweighed the slight increase in cost of the laparoscopic procedure itself. This was a very detailed paper. Forty-nine of his procedures were for biopsy of intra-abdominal malignancies. Not only was he well ahead of his time in terms of health economics, he was also a physician already moving in on his colleagues' surgical domain. Does this have an echo in the present time? Veress (1938), an innovative surgeon from Hungary, introduced the spring-loaded insufflation needle which is little different from the one we use routinely today. Further changes in laparoscopy were slow to be reported, probably because of the continued criticism by fellow physicians and surgeons.

The controlled automatic insufflator was introduced by Semm (Fig. 2.1) in the late 1960s, and it is Semm himself (1978, 1982a, 1982b, 1983, 1986, 1989) who began to describe the more elaborate operative procedures that most of the gynaecological world seemed to choose to ignore until the late 1980s. It is interesting to see that Semm's work, which also included the first reported laparoscopic appendicectomy (Semm 1983), once heavily criticized even by gynaecologists and general surgeons in Germany, has now received a fresh appraisal. As a living father of this technology, his presence is in even greater demand around the world.

However, the catalyst for the explosion of interest in operative laparoscopy focuses on the laparoscopic cholecystectomy. This was first reported by Dubois *et al.* (1989) who then went on to describe three years of experience of this technique in 1990. On the other side of the Atlantic, Reddick *et al.* (1989) reported on his series of over 200 laparoscopic cholecystectomies when most other surgeons were still arguing over the theoretical advantages. Reddick began to convince his colleagues, and more importantly the public, that laparoscopic techniques were the way ahead.

It is difficult to understand the very rapid acceptance of these techniques by both clinicians and patients in the last five years, but it probably reflects improved communication and health education. As a prime example of minimally invasive surgery, laparoscopy not only benefits the patient in terms of a more rapid return to normal activities and reduced morbidity but also benefits those who control our health economy. There has been an undeniable interest from government officials, hospital administrators and politicians in such techniques and this has again reinforced the public's awareness. What has been in the melting pot for 92 years has now snowballed with rapidly gaining momentum, and each new publication from each newly formed journal brings yet another innovative step to refine further the techniques of laparoscopy and expand its horizons.

Several urologists have been involved in the development of laparoscopy in the last 10 years. Eshghi *et al.* (1985) described a percutaneous transperitoneal laparoscopic approach to a pelvic kidney and subsequent endoscopic removal of a staghorn calculus. Das & Amar (1988) and Whitfield & Ryan (1990) also discussed the potential for

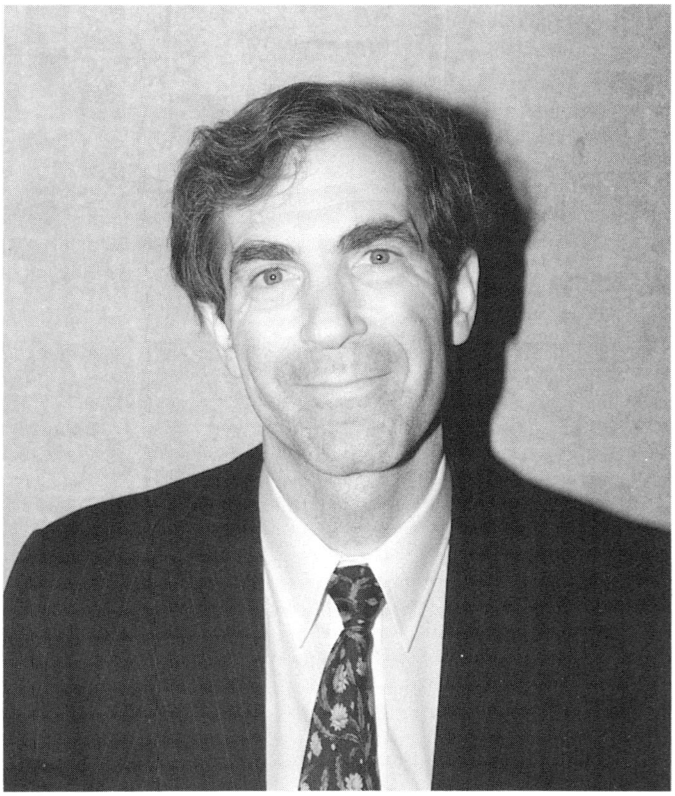

Fig. 2.2 Professor Ralph Clayman, St Louis, USA. In 1991 he performed the first laparoscopic nephrectomy.

laparoscopic techniques in urology, but the greatest credit must always go to Ralph Clayman (Fig. 2.2), who not has only made enormous contributions to endourology as a whole, but developed many of the more complicated techniques such as a laparoscopic nephrectomy (Clayman *et al.* 1991), and then convinced the rest of us that this was the way ahead.

References

Bernheim B.M. (1911) Organoscopy: Cystoscopy of the abdominal cavity. *Annals of Surgery*, **53**, 764.

Clayman R., Kavoussi L., Soper N. *et al.* (1991) Laparoscopic nephrectomy: Initial case report. *Journal of Urology*, **146**, 278–82.

Das S. & Amar A.D. The impact of laparoscopy on modern urological practice. *Urological Clinics of North America*, **15**: 3, 537–40.

Dubois F., Berthelot G., Levard H. (1989) Cholecystectomie par coelioscopie. *Nouvelle presse médicale*, **18**, 980–2.

Dubois F., Icard P., Berthelot G., Levard H. (1990) Coelioscopic cholecystectomy. *Annals of Surgery*, **211**, 60–2.

Eshghi A.M., Roth J.S., Smith A.D. (1985) Percutaneous transperitoneal approach to a pelvic kidney for endourological removal of a staghorn calculus. *Journal of Urology*, **134**, 525–7.

Fervers C. (1933) Die Laparoskopie mit dem Zystokope. Ein Beitrag zur Vereinfachung der Technik und zur endoskopischen Strangdurchtrennung in der Bauchole. *Medizinische Klinik*, **29**, 1042–5.

Jacobeus H.C. (1910) Über die Möglichkeiten, die Zystoskopie bei Untersuchung seroser Hohlungen anzuwenden. *Münchener medezinische Wochenschrift*, **57**, 2090–2.

Kelling G. (1901) Über Ösophagoskopie, Gastroskopie und Colioskopie. *Münchener medezinische Wochenschrift*, **49**, 21–4.

Nordentöft S. (1912) Über Endoskopie geschlossener Kavitaten mittels meines Trokar-Endoskopes. *Verhandlungen der Deutchen Gesellschaft für Gynakologie*, **41**, 78-81.

Ott D. (1901) Illumination of the abdomen (ventroscopia) (Russian). *Journal Akuschezologii Zhenskoi*, **15**, 1045.

Reddick E.J., Olsen D., Daniell J., Saye W. *et al.* (1989) Laparoscopic laser cholecystectomy. *Lasers in Medicine and Surgery*, February, 38–40.

Ruddock J.C. (1937) Peritoneoscopy. *Surgery, Gynaecology and Obstetrics*, **65**, 623.

Semm K. (1978) Tissue puncher and loop ligation. New aids for surgical therapeutic pelviscopy (laparoscopy): Endoscopic intra-abdominal surgery. *Endoscopy*, **10**, 119–27.

Semm K. (1982a) Advances in pelviscopic surgery (appendicectomy) *Current Problems in Obstetrics, Gynaecology and Fertility*, **5** (10).

Semm K. (1982b) The endoscopic intra-abdominal suture. *Geburtshilfe und Frauenheilkunde*, **42**, 56–7.

Semm K. (1983) Endoscopic appendicectomy. *Endoscopy*, **15**, 59–64.

Semm K. (1986) Operative pelviscopy. *British Medical Bulletin*, **42**, 284–95.

Semm K. (1989) History. In: *Operative Gynaecologic Endoscopy* (eds J.S. Sanfillipo & R.L. Levine). Springer-Verlag, New York.

Stolkind E.J. (1919) The value of pleuroscopy (thoracoscopy) in the diagnosis of pulmonary diseases and laparoscopy in the diagnosis of abdominal diseases. *The Medical Press*, 1 January.

Veress J. (1938) Neues Instrument zur Ausführung von Brust oder Bauchpunktionen. *Deutsche medizinische Wochenschrift*, 41, 1480–1.

Whitfield H.N., Ryan K.J. (1990) Experimental laparoscopic surgery: potential clinical applications in urology. *Journal of Endourology*, **4**: 1, 37–47.

Zollikofer R. (1925) Zur Laparoskopie. *Schweizerische medizinische Wochenschrift*, **5**, 264–5.

3: Instrumentation

M.J. COPTCOAT AND C.G. EDEN

Telescopes

One of the most significant advances in rigid endoscopy was the development of the rod lens system in 1966 by the British optical physicist Hopkins. His design, which utilizes air spaces for the lenses, resulted in vastly improved image brightness and clarity. Most of the endoscope manufacturers now use a hybrid of this system, and contrary to popular opinion amongst urologists, there is a great deal of difference between the different manufacturers' telescopes. The rigid endoscope consists of an objective lens, relay lens, eye piece lens and illumination light guide. The eye piece lens has an approximate magnification of $\times$ 3 and this could be easily increased for future endoscopic microsurgical work.

The field of view varies with each manufacturer's endoscope. The 'field of view' describes the area observable from the tip of the endoscope. The greater the field of view, the greater the area that can be observed, given that the distance from the lens is the same. If the visual field is merely widened, the image will become smaller. The 'observed field of view' refers to the size of the visual field observed through the rigid endoscope, thus the larger the observed field of view, the larger the image (Fig. 3.1). The 'direction of view' (Fig. 3.2) refers to the angle between the centre of the visual field and the longitudinal axis of the endoscope. Standard laparoscopes have a 0° or 30°

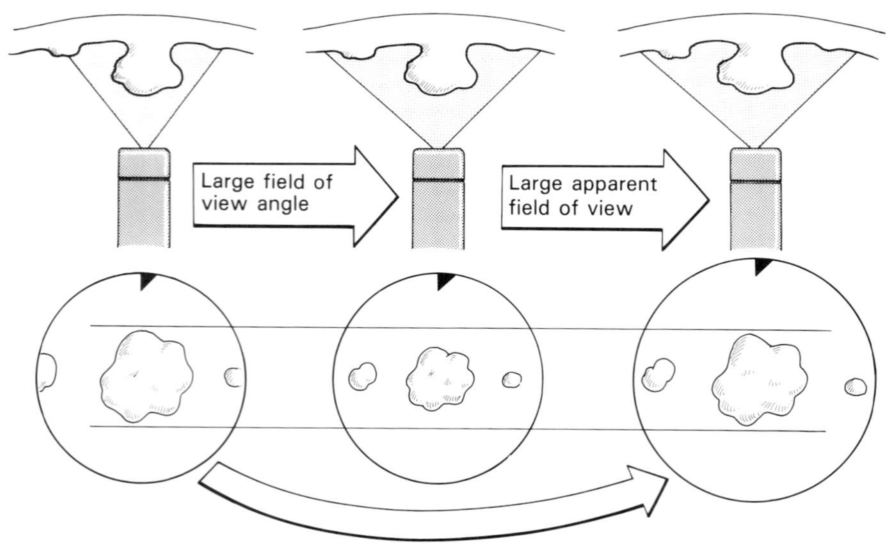

Fig. 3.1 Field of view and apparent field of view in rigid laparoscopes vary with each manufacturer's endoscope. The greater the field of view, the greater the area that can be observed. If the visual field is merely widened, the image will become smaller. The larger the 'observed field of view', the larger the image.

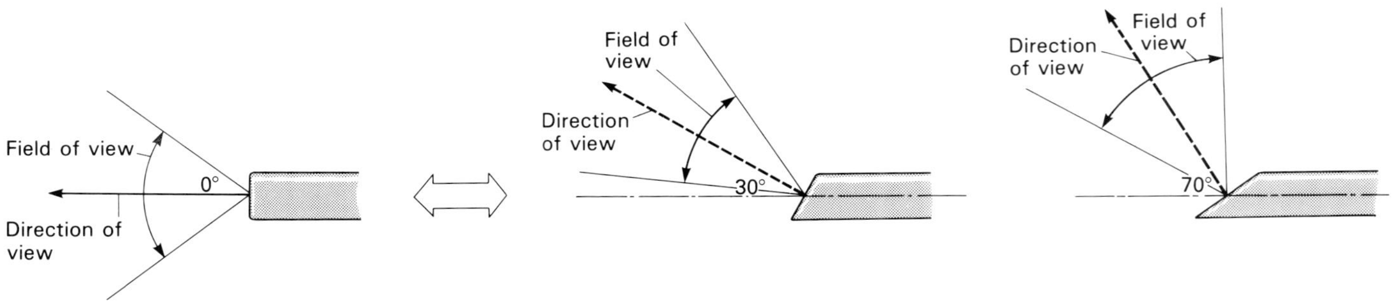

Fig. 3.2 Direction of view and field of view of a laparoscope. The 'direction of view' refers to the angle between the centre of the visual field and the longitudinal axis of the endoscope.

direction of view but we will probably see the introduction of increased angles for specific complex manoeuvres. Endoscopic instrument orientation is easiest when visualized through a 0° telescope but one sometimes has a restricted view of the site of dissection and a different direction of view can help the operator to see over obstacles. The disadvantage in instrument orientation is then of secondary importance.

The overall diameter of the telescopes used in laparoscopy is approximately 9 mm and they require a 10 mm port. Telescopes are available with an integrated working channel. The presence of such a working channel usually reduces the diameter and therefore the clarity of the lens image, and using manipulative devices in this way is usually confined to simple manoeuvres such as the clipping of Fallopian tubes. They do not really have a place in more complex operative laparoscopy where more sensitive instrument orientation is required.

One of the greatest practical problems during prolonged operative laparoscopy is misting of the objective lens within the abdomen. This occurs because of the relative imbalance between intraperitoneal temperatures and the temperature of the telescope. It is exacerbated by the use of diathermy or lasers near the lens.

Up until now, the only ways to deal with this have been the repeated removal and warming of the telescope in hot water or the use of demisting solutions. Even the latter solution requires removal of the telescope every 10–15 minutes. This can be very tedious during a complex manoeuvre. Some manufacturers have recently introduced a telescope with its own irrigating and self-cleaning lens. Whilst this has added bulk to the telescope it has proved to be one way around an otherwise irritating problem.

Cameras

Coptcoat spent some time with Professor Semm in Kiel, Germany, in 1988. Semm had been carrying out operative laparoscopy since 1973, and 97% of his routine gynaecological workload was then carried out

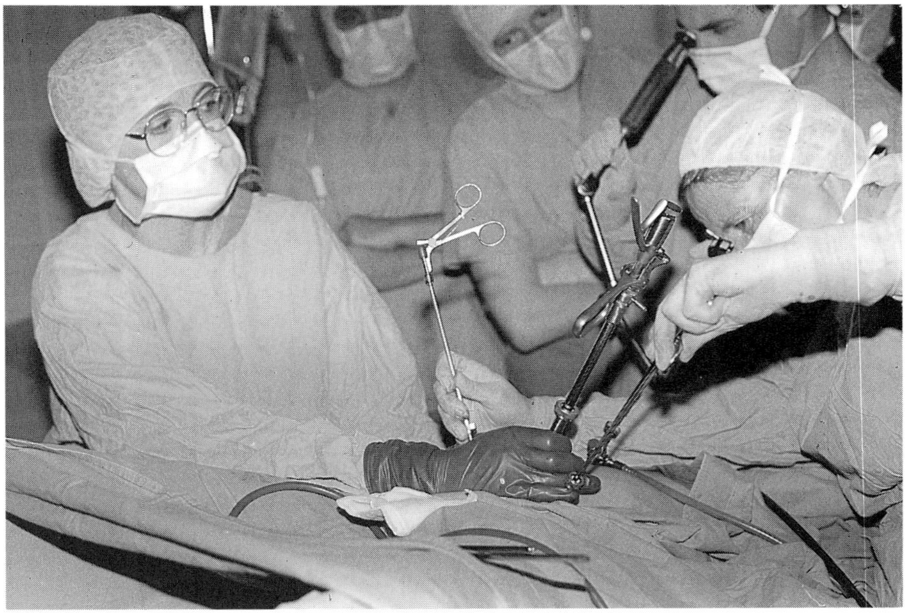

Fig 3.3 Complex operative laparoscopy in Kiel in 1989, without the benefit of the video camera.

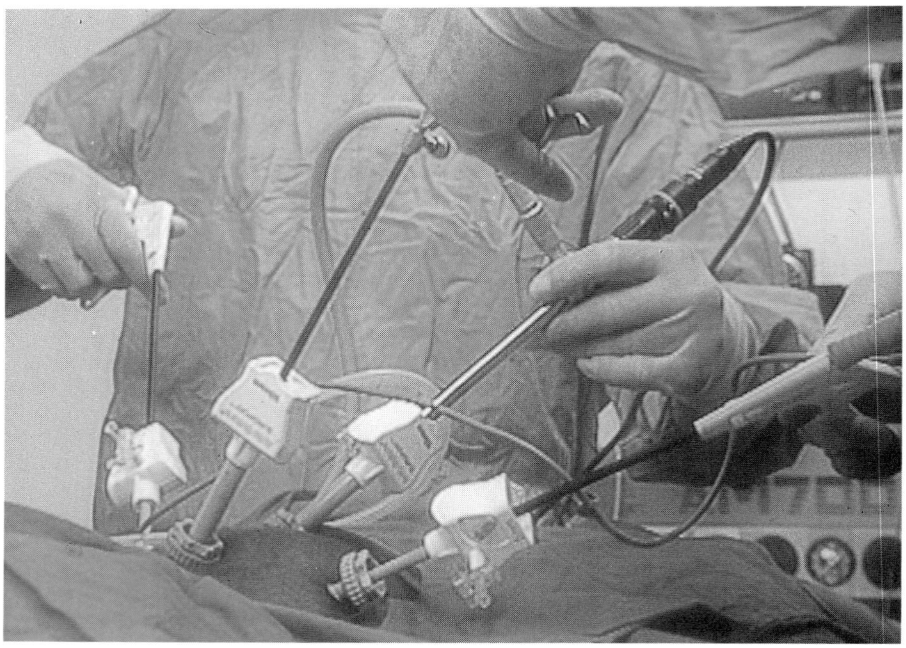

Fig 3.4 Complex operative laparoscopy in London in 1993.

laparoscopically. Coptcoat was able to witness the need for multiple theatres because of the increased operative time, but one small observation stood out more than the rest and this was the requirement of gymnastic qualities by the primary operators (Fig. 3.3).

At this time, video cameras were not in use and the operator had to keep his or her eye close to the telescope whilst moving instruments at full arm's length. Whilst one is welcome to carry on in this way, the advent of laparoscopic cholecystectomy performed using the video camera has introduced an indirect and ergonomically more

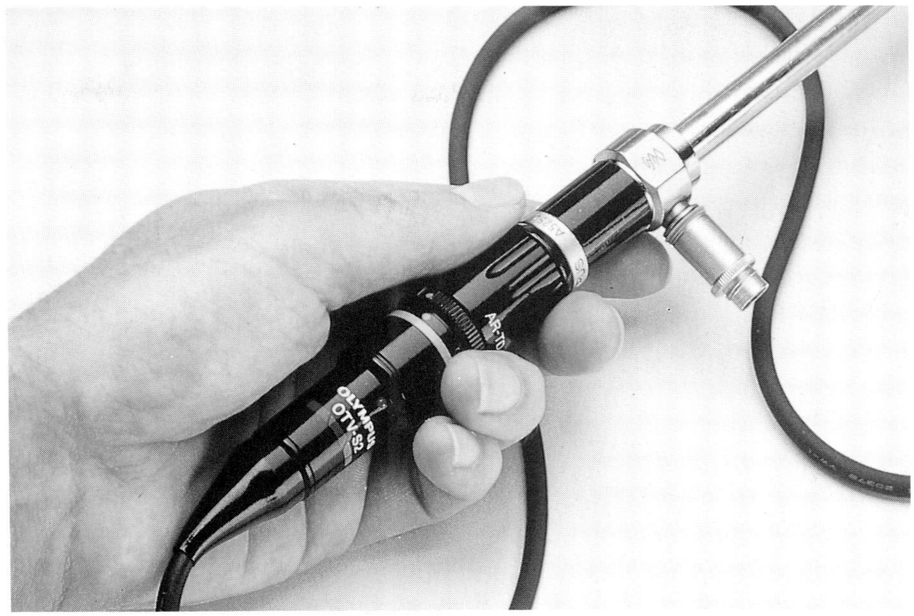

Fig. 3.5 A high-quality CCD camera used for operative laparoscopy.

Table 3.1 Imaging systems tested at King's College Hospital, London

Camera	Light source	Telescope
GU-8001	8003	8011
Olympus OTV-S2	CLV-10	A5254A
Olympus OTV-S4	CLV-10	A5254A
Storz 9050PB	450DV	26033AP
Wolf 5500.11	5130	8934.441

pleasing type of surgery to most of our departments. Operating whilst watching a video monitor (Fig. 3.4) is a new and initially demanding experience with its own learning curve. However, most of us as urologists should be familiar with this if we are carrying out our prostatic resections in a similar way.

The modern charge-coupled device (CCD) camera (Fig. 3.5) is an essential requirement for teaching and training and its routine use will allow us to make the step into operative laparoscopy with much less difficulty. The camera should be handed to a urologist whenever any form of endoscopy is taking place.

There are many CCD cameras on the market at present, and we have carried out an objective assessment of five of these systems. The optical design and image quality were assessed using an optical bench, a Sony UP5000 colour videoprinter and three test cards. Vertical, horizontal and rotational scales on the optical bench were set to zero before the telescope was clamped in position with its window 45mm from the test target.

The light source output was set to automatic and the image was colour-balanced. The target was manually focused using the central part of the test grid (KeyMed 1992). Each set of videoprints was examined by an independent optical engineer without knowledge of the corresponding imaging system and was assessed with regard to optical design, image quality, illumination and colour rendition.

There was a surprisingly large and dramatic difference in the optical performance of the imaging systems tested. Whilst the performance of some was disappointing, two of these systems produced images with excellent resolution, brightness and colour rendition: the GU-8001 camera, 8003 light source and 8011 telescope; and the Olympus OTV-S4 camera, CLV-10 light source and A5254A telescope combination.

Of the two, the GU system produced an image with considerable distortion, field curvature and moderate astigmatism, whereas the Olympus system produced a flat image with no distortion and only very slight astigmatism.

The optics of the Olympus OTV-S4 CCD camera, when used with the CLV-10 light source and A5254A telescope, are superior to the other systems tested and provide an image with good resolution, brightness and colour rendition. Interestingly, only the two Olympus systems produced an image free of distortion or field curvature and with very slight astigmatism. This is clearly a great asset in operative laparoscopy, in which depth perception is always difficult because of the two-dimensional image provided.

The other significant visual handicap in operative laparoscopy is the left-to-right inverted image on the first assistant's monitor when two monitors are being used, as in a laparoscopic nephrectomy. Great patience on the part of the operator and careful practice on the part of the assistant are necessary!

Current developments in CCD technology include improved light sensitivity (increased pixels), better colour rendition (three-chip cameras) and the use of three-dimensional imaging systems. 3-D cameras are now available but are very bulky and expensive; we all eagerly await their refinement because of the dramatic effect it will have on our endocoordination.

The routine use of an imaging system in endourology (O'Boyle 1990) reduces the possibility of contact with potentially contaminated body fluids, fatigue and, ultimately, operating time. It increases image size, accuracy and comfort as well as interest in the operation by theatre staff and is also an ideal teaching aid. Its routine use in endourology enables the neolaparoscopist to improve endocoordination and orientation before embarking on operative laparoscopy with which he will then rapidy become comfortable.

Insufflators

The artificial space within the peritoneal cavity is achieved and maintained by filling with a gas that distends the abdominal wall. This is termed the pneumoperitoneum.

In the history of laparoscopy, many gases have been used for establishing a pneumoperitoneum, including room air, nitrous oxide, oxygen and carbon dioxide. Air and oxygen create a higher risk in terms of air embolism. In addition, they support combustion, which is dangerous when using electrocautery or laser energy. Nitrous oxide has unpredictable effects because of its rapid absorption into the blood stream. Nitrous oxide was commonly used for diagnostic laparoscopy but because the gas also supports combustion, its use tends to preclude any dissection.

Carbon dioxide has therefore become the standard gas used for creating a pneumoperitoneum. It is relatively safe in that it can be injected directly into the blood stream in volumes up to 100 ml per minute without serious metabolic effects. It also suppresses combustion. This is all very fortunate because carbon dioxide is also the most readily available and inexpensive gas.

A modern insufflator (see Fig. 3.6) is now a piece of sophisticated equipment that has been developed to deliver carbon dioxide automatically from a high-pressured pressure tank through a regulator and into the patient at predetermined flow rates. These machines constantly monitor the intra-abdominal pressure and stop the flow once a certain pressure is reached.

They usually indicate the rate of flow and record the total volume of gas delivered from the machine. Rapid insufflation into the abdomen is necessary when there is a leak around a valve or during the exchange of instruments. Therefore, operative laparoscopic surgery requires a high-flow insufflator capable of delivering at least 6 l of gas per minute. The new machines are set with an upper pressure limit of 15 mm of mercury. It is safer to work at a pressure of 10 mm of mercury during procedures that last several hours. A lower

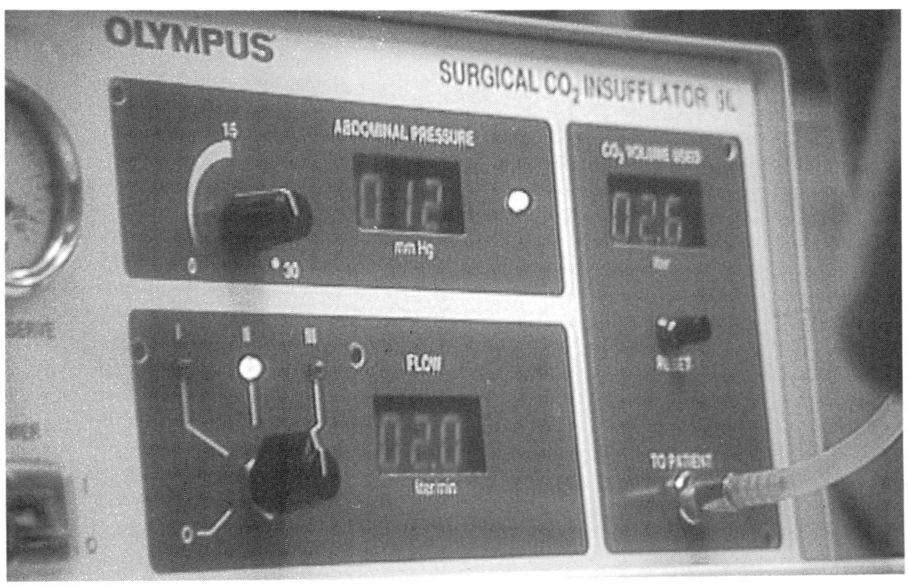

Fig 3.6 A modern, automatic high-flow carbon dioxide insufflator used in operative laparoscopy.

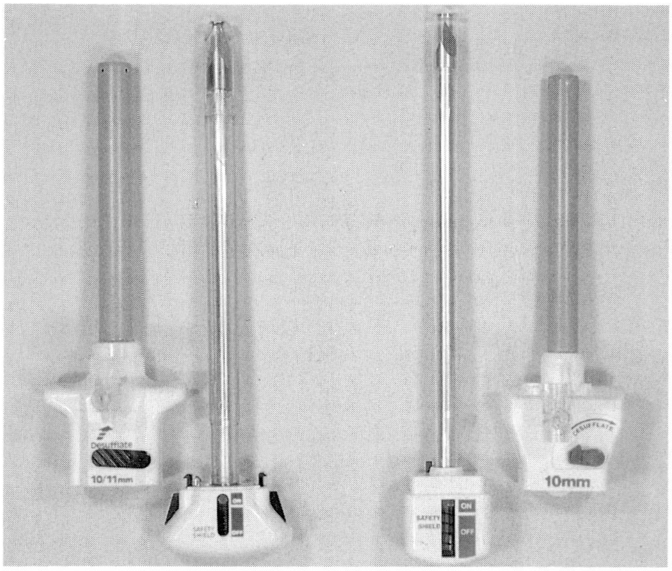

Fig. 3.7

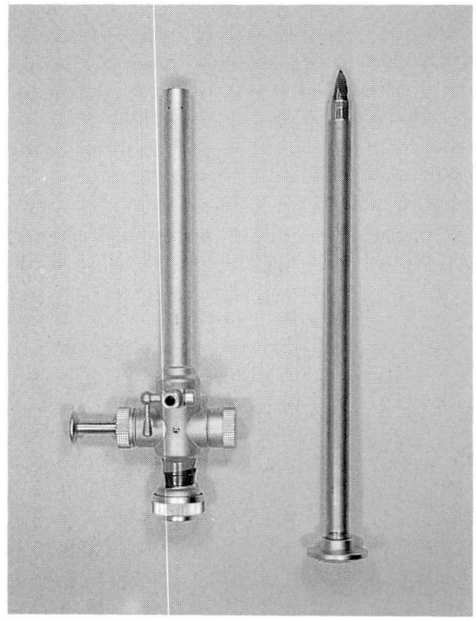

Fig. 3.8

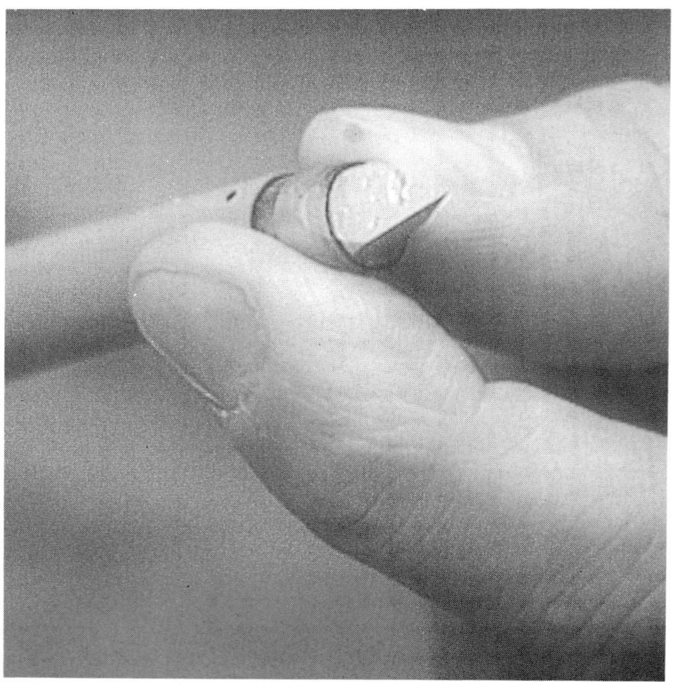

Fig. 3.9

Fig. 3.7 Two disposable laparoscopic ports, each consisting of a trocar, with safety shield, and cannula.

Fig. 3.8 A nondisposable laparoscopic port, consisting of a trocar and cannula.

Fig. 3.9 The retractable safety shield at the tip of a disposable laparoscope port is held back in this view. The shield covers the sharp trocar as soon as it enters the peritoneum.

intra-abdominal pressure seems to produce less haemodynamic instability, prevent congestion of low-pressure venous capillary beds and certainly does not splint the diaphragm to any great extent.

Ports

The term 'port' has has come into use to refer to the combination of

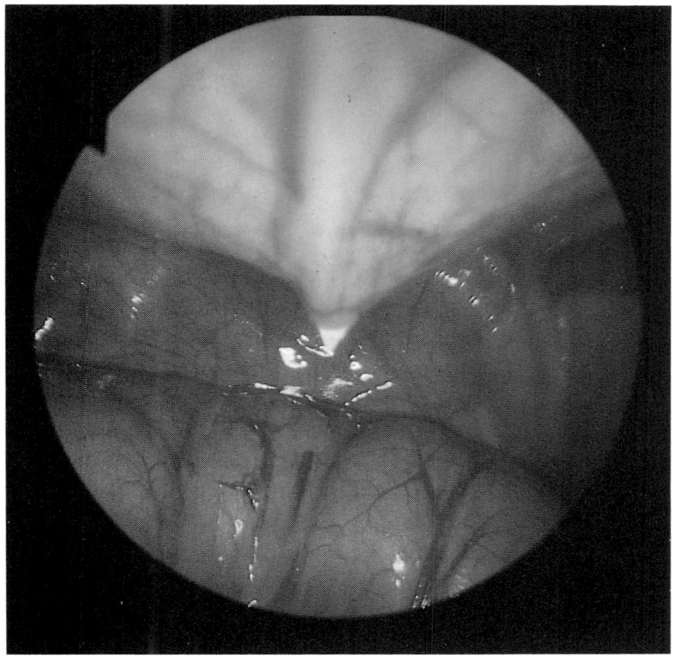

Fig. 3.10 An endopscopic view showing the sharp trocar of the disposable port penetrating the peritoneum.

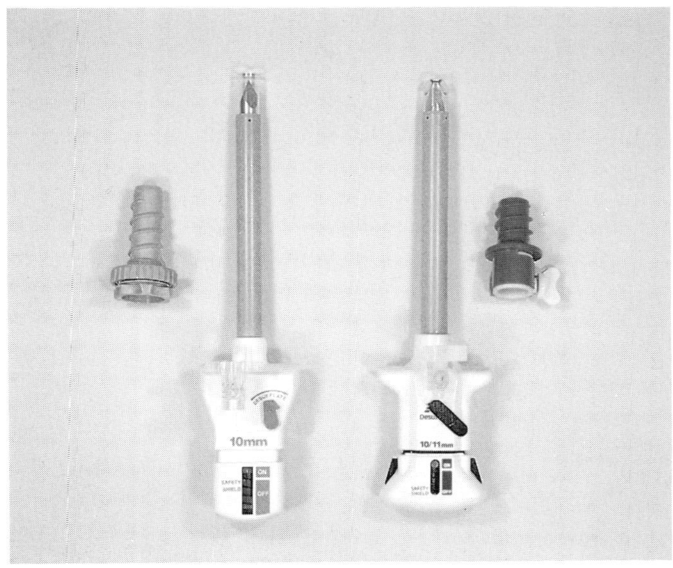

Fig. 3.11 Grips can be used to hold the laparoscopic port within the muscle fascia.

trocar and cannula. There are both nondisposable and disposable ports (Figs 3.7, 3.8). Flap valves, which are found almost exclusively in disposable ports, are superior to trumpet valves which tend to strip diathermy insulation off hand instruments. They also allow easier insertion of instruments, and the insertion of instruments single-handed.

The advantages of the flap valve, together with the incorporation of a retractable safety shield (Figs 3.9, 3.10) to cover the trocar tip once it has penetrated the peritoneum, justifies the routine use of disposable ports for the primary or telescope port at least. If finances are limited, the use of a disposable primary port and nondisposable secondary ports is a relatively inexpensive but safe compromise. The use of tissue grips on all ports to prevent inadvertant displacement is essential in all but diagnostic laparoscopic procedures (Fig. 3.11).

Probably the most important decision to be made is whether to use disposable or reusable ports and hand instruments or to compromise and to use a mixture. This has very considerable cost implications. For example, the extra cost of disposable equipment necessary to perform a laparoscopic varicocelectomy and a laparoscopic nephrectomy at 1992 prices is £417 and £917 respectively. This cost can be considerably reduced by using certain 'essential' disposables (such as the Veress needle, primary port and insulated scissors) in conjunction with reusable equipment.

Although the overriding arbiter is often budget, other important factors are reliability, instrument performance (such as scissor or trocar sharpness) and handling, potential for cross-patient contamination and ease of cleaning. Whether choosing disposable or reusable equipment, the best advice is to spend as much money as is available and to buy only good-quality instruments.

A Hasson blunt-tipped port (Fig. 3.12) (see Chapter 4, General laparoscopic techniques) is essential when previous abdominal scars suggest adhesions. A nondisposable type is recommended, because a safety shield is not required.

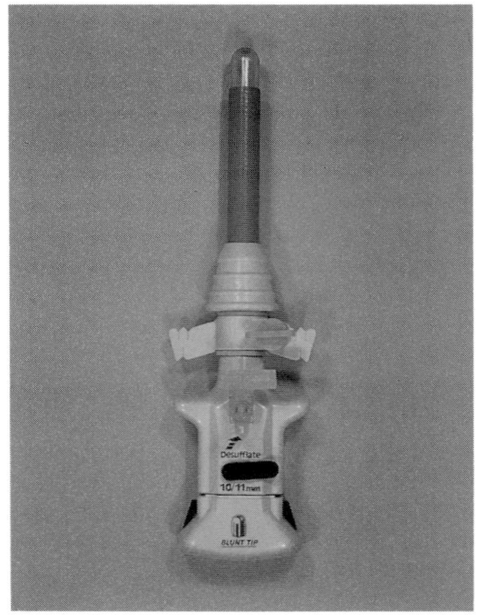

Fig. 3.12 A Hasson blunt-tipped port can be introduced by a minilaparotomy incision when abdominal scars suggest adhesions.

Manipulative instruments

The variety of manipulative instruments for laparoscopy is increasing all the time, and each new conference sees the introduction of an even greater variety. In many cases we are seeing the conversion of standard open manipulative instruments to a size and form suitable for laparoscopy. The small surface area of contact on tissues allowed for each of these instruments means that their roles are much more specific.

It is now possible to obtain a wide variety of tissue-holding forceps, retractors, dissection instruments, needle-holders and probes (Figs 3.13–3.15).

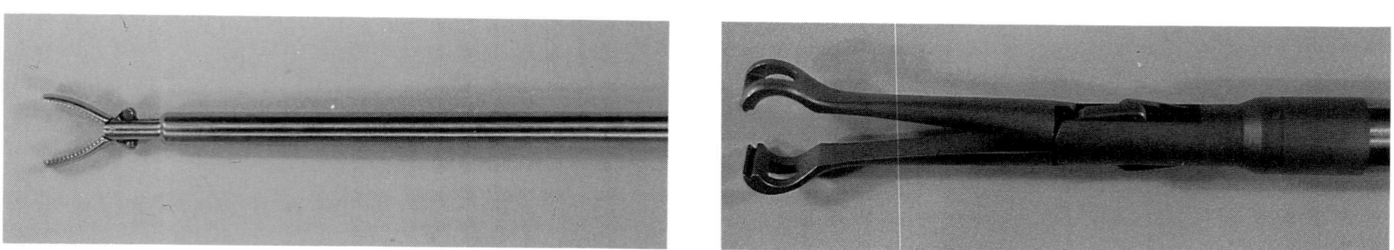

(a) (b)

Fig. 3.13 Laparoscopic forceps: (a) soft-tissue forceps, (b) Babcock forceps.

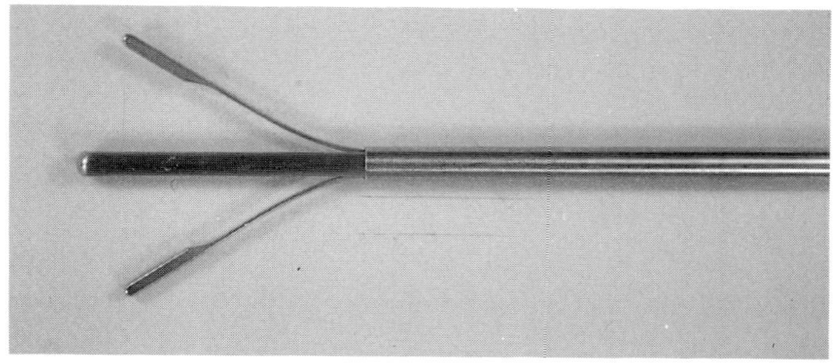

Fig. 3.14 A laparoscopic fan retractor.

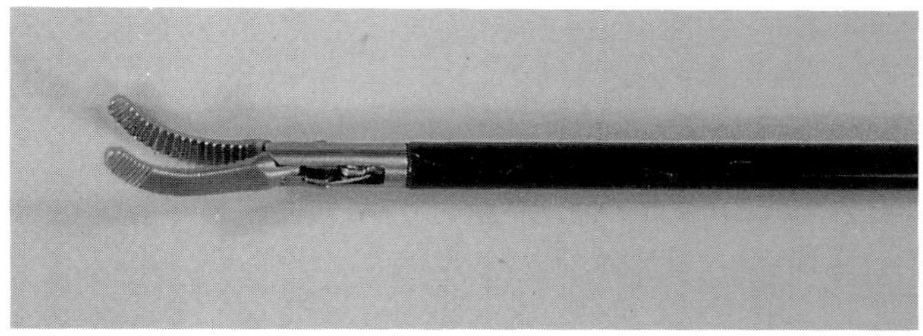

Fig. 3.15 A laparoscopic curved dissector.

One of the great difficulties in operative laparoscopy is the retraction of tissues away from the site of operation. One does not have the benefits of the size 8 assistant's hand nor a wet pack under a ring retractor. It is the introduction of various ingenious retraction devices that is now allowing us to carry out much more complex laparoscopic surgery in urology.

We have carried out an objective assessment of various laparoscopic manipulation instruments.

The handle-closure force needed to produce a 1 kg force at the jaws of five instruments of varying design with conventional handles (Fig. 3.16) was measured. This was achieved using two opposed spring balances applied to the handle blades and a calibrated force transducer between the instrument's jaws. The force needed to open the jaws of two spring-handled instruments was also measured by applying a

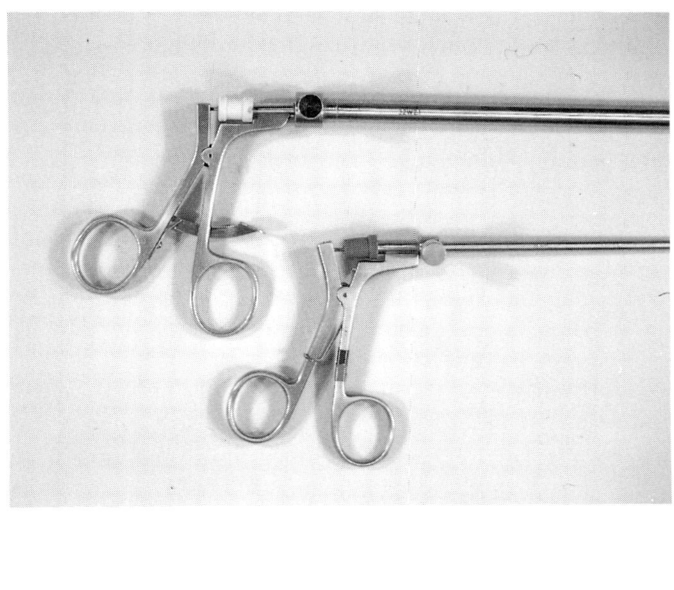

Fig. 3.16 Two conventional designs for instrument handles: ratchet-adjusted (top) and spring-handled (bottom).

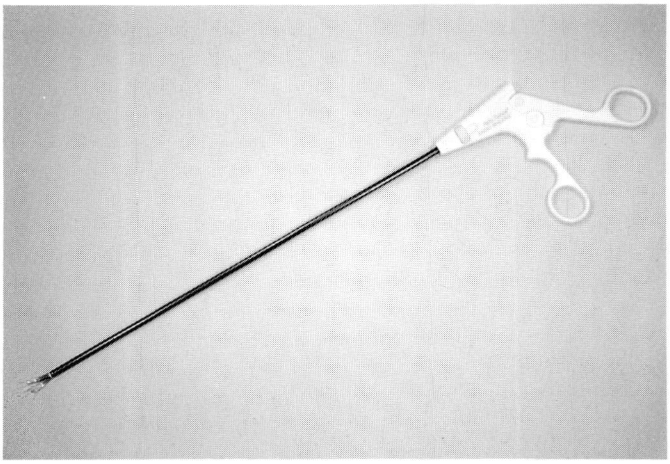

Fig. 3.17 Disposable laparoscopic endoshears. They are sharp and insulated for monopolar diathermy application. To prevent unnecessary blunting of the blades, diathermy should only be applied through closed shears.

force to the spring while the instrument was resting on electronic scales. Additionally, we measured the closure force needed to cut a single piece of paper (80 gsm) with two scissors (one fine-curved and one heavy-hooked) using a spring balance. Each experiment was repeated three times.

There was no significant difference in mechanical advantage (force generated at the jaws or force applied to the handles) amongst the conventionally-handled instruments. Instruments with a variety of handle designs, incorporating different ratchet systems were examined; including conventional scissor-pattern handle (for use with forearm in neutral or supinated positions); spring handle; pistol grip and pen grip.

The handle design *per se* was felt to be unimportant functionally but the design of the ratchet significantly influenced the ease of operation, particularly when held in the nondominant hand. Although they required the greatest force to open the jaws, spring-handled instruments were the easiest to release. The horizontal ratchet was the most difficult to release with the vertical ratchet falling between the two.

Extra-short instruments were often found to be too short unless the ports were sited immediately over the operation site, which in turn often made for a more difficult dissection. The use of extra-long instruments produced an exaggerated shake artefact and resulted in clumsier tissue manipulation.

As there is no significant difference in mechanical advantage amongst the conventionally handled instruments, the final choice depends very much on the feel of the instrument, the features offered (especially the facility for diathermy), user-friendliness and budget. Our preference for the dominant hand is for instruments which are insulated and have rotatable shafts. Operating a ratchet with the non-dominant hand is awkward and slow and we recommend the use of spring-handled grasping forceps for this task.

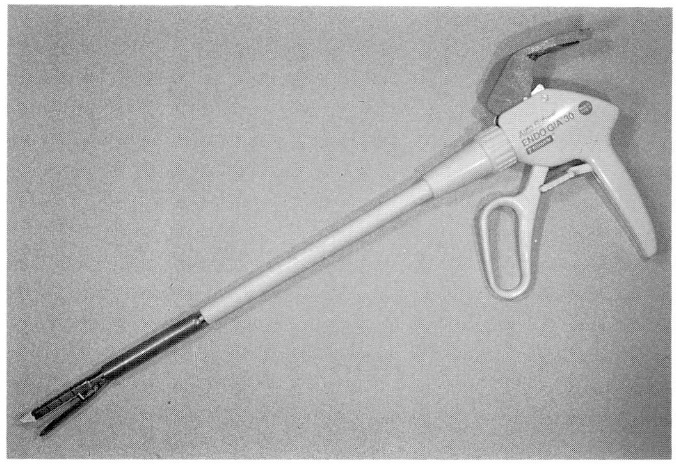

Fig. 3.18 The Endo GIA* 30 stapler and incisor. It provides secure haemostasis for blood vessels greater than 5 mm in diameter.

The use of disposable diathermy scissors (Fig. 3.17) ensures predictable, efficient and precise cutting and aids fast and accurate dissection, and this is probably the only essential disposable manipulative instrument.

Sutures

Semm pioneered the technique of laparoscopic suturing. He employed this for the re-anastomosis of a Fallopian tube, using a 2/0 gauge catgut on a short 1 cm straight needle. There are now many more sutures available for use with laparoscopic needle-holders.

In particular, there is a selection of sutures available from Ethicon which utilize a quarter-curved needle called the Ski needle. This has the advantage that it can be introduced through a 5 mm laparoscopic port but also is curved enough to be an aid to anastomotic suturing. All types of suture material have been made available by Ethicon with this round-bodied needle.

Laparoscopic suturing can be quite time-consuming and there are many instances, particularly with regard to small-bowel anastomoses, when the Endo GIA 30 stapler (Fig. 3.18) is much faster and just as safe. This instrument from AutoSuture is available in a 3 cm form, thus requiring at least two applications to provide a suitable anastomotic lumen; a 6 cm cartridge is due to be introduced in the near future. Similar staplers will soon be available from Ethicon. At the present time, a small-bowel re-anastomosis during the formation of an ileal conduit requires at least 4 fires of the Endo GIA 30 stapler.

Haemostatic devices

Monopolar diathermy current used from either the dissecting scissors

*A trademark of the United States Surgical Corporation (AutoSuture).

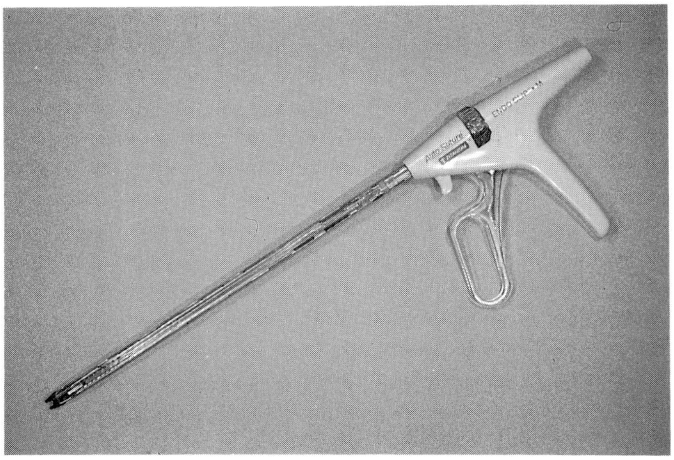

Fig. 3.19 A disposable Endoclip Applier. To achieve secure haemostasis, it is important to visualize the opposing clip ends across a well-dissected vessel .

or separate laparoscopic forceps is a method commonly employed for vessels up to 2mm in diameter. Beyond this, and certainly for arterial haemostasis, one requires mechanical clipping devices. Three sorts are available and these have been evaluated in our department by Eden and Popert.

The recent enthusiasm for laparoscopic surgery has resulted in the development and refinement of a variety of mechanical haemostatic devices. To date, there are no guidelines for the use of these devices. Eden's and Popert's study establishes such guidelines and has considerable cost implications.

A series of bursting pressure-vessel diameter curves were constructed using mesenteric arteries of two-year-old sheep and three commercially available occlusive devices. The haemostatic devices assessed were:

1 Medium-large Endoclip Applier (AutoSuture) (Fig. 3.19)
2 Lockable PDS AP400 clip (Ethicon)
3 Endo GIA 30 stapler (AutoSuture)

The bursting pressure was measured for each device on arteries with external diameters of 3mm, 5mm, 7mm and 9mm. Each experiment was conducted using static and pulsatile flow and was repeated at least three times.

All three devices could be applied securely up to a vessel diameter of 5mm, withstanding a pressure of 500cmH_2O. Beyond this diameter, the clip did not totally occlude the vessel lumen.

The maximum diameter vessel which could be accommodated in the jaws of the PDS clip was 7mm. The vessel withstood a pressure of 500cmH_2O. The Endo GIA 30 stapler occluded vessels of all sizes and also withstood a pressure of 500cmH_2O. The clips can be applied safely to vessels up to 5mm in diameter and they are provided in a multifire cartridge.

Lockable PDS AP400 clips should be used for larger vessels up to 7mm in diameter, but have the practical disadvantage of having to be loaded singly. The use of the Endo GIA 30 stapler should be reserved for vessels greater than 7 mm in diameter, such as renal artery and vein.

Water-jet dissectors

Semm was the first to introduce a combined instrument for saline irrigation and aspiration. This instrument is very helpful for removing small amounts of blood. However, it is necessary always to remember that during aspiration, the tip of the probe must be kept under the fluid level or you will witness a rapid decompression of the pneumoperitoneum.

Many companies have increased the pressure of irrigation and termed the new inspiration a dissector. The concept is that the probe is then placed in the subperitoneal tissues and the reflux of saline dissects away the fat leaving the vessels and other structures free.

These modifications have not always been helpful, because the resultant tissues can be much more difficult to manipulate. Without doubt we will see such instruments refined in the near future, for they do hold great promise.

Lasers and diathermy

There was a great debate during the advent of the laparoscopic cholecystectomy as to whether laser or diathermy dissection was more efficient and safer. This was an argument fuelled by several laser companies who saw that their sales had been dwindling and expected a new market to open up to them, especially if they donated a laser to key clinicians.

The Nd:YAG laser combined with a sapphire tip has never been anything other than an expensive form of monopolar diathermy and both can be used for dissection and coagulation of vessels up to 1 mm in diameter without any coaptation. Using either of these energy forms for dissection causes unnecessary local increases in heat and misting of the telescope, and endoscopic scissors with diathermy, directed through the scissors, are greatly to be preferred when small vessels are visually encountered. This enables a much cleaner form of dissection. It is important to keep the scissors closed when using diathermy to prevent blunting when the current takes the route of least resistance across the sharp blade.

Retrieval devices

These are in essence simple impermeable bags (Fig. 3.21) which are used to collect organs and tissue within the abdomen and bring them safely onto the abdominal wall via one of the ports (Fig. 3.22). They

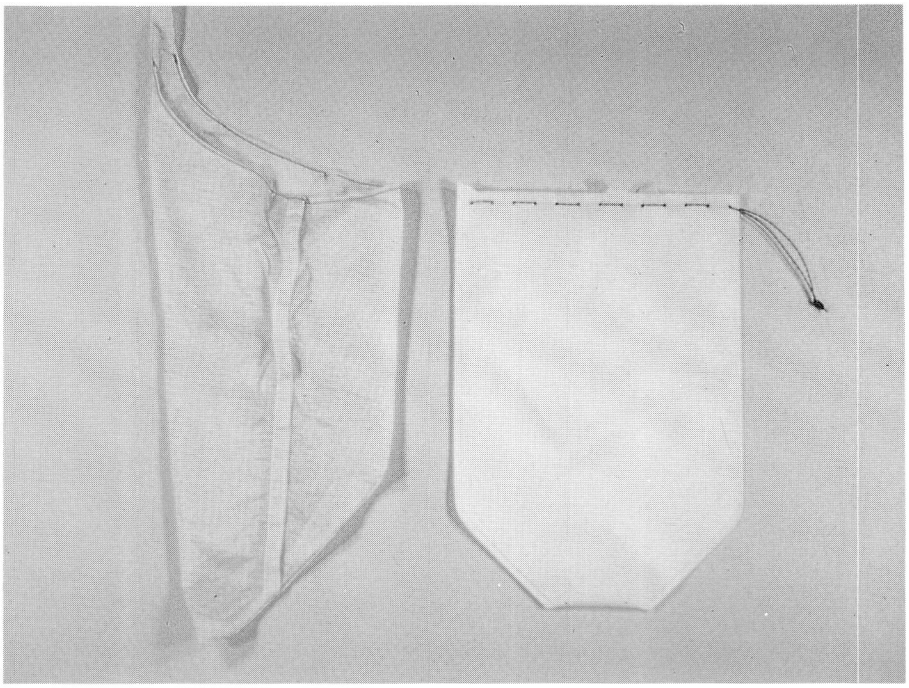

Fig. 3.20 Two designs of kidney retrieval bag. The bags are impermeable to cellular fluid and are made of rip-proof nylon.

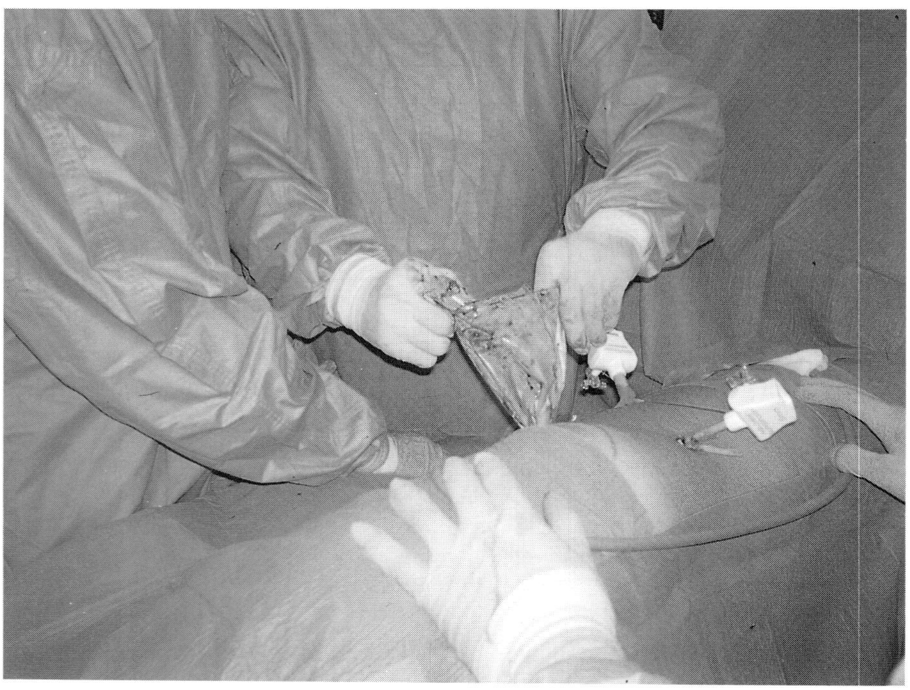

Fig. 3.21 The neck of the retrieval bag has been brought out on to the abdominal wall during a nephrectomy, prior to morcellation within the bag.

were first introduced for infected or 'hot' gall bladders but are now used for the removal of bowel tumours and end organs such as the ovary, kidney and spleen.

They are much more than just a bag in that they must be of such a design that can be easily introduced through a port and be strong enough to withstand the morcellation that is required when tissue is

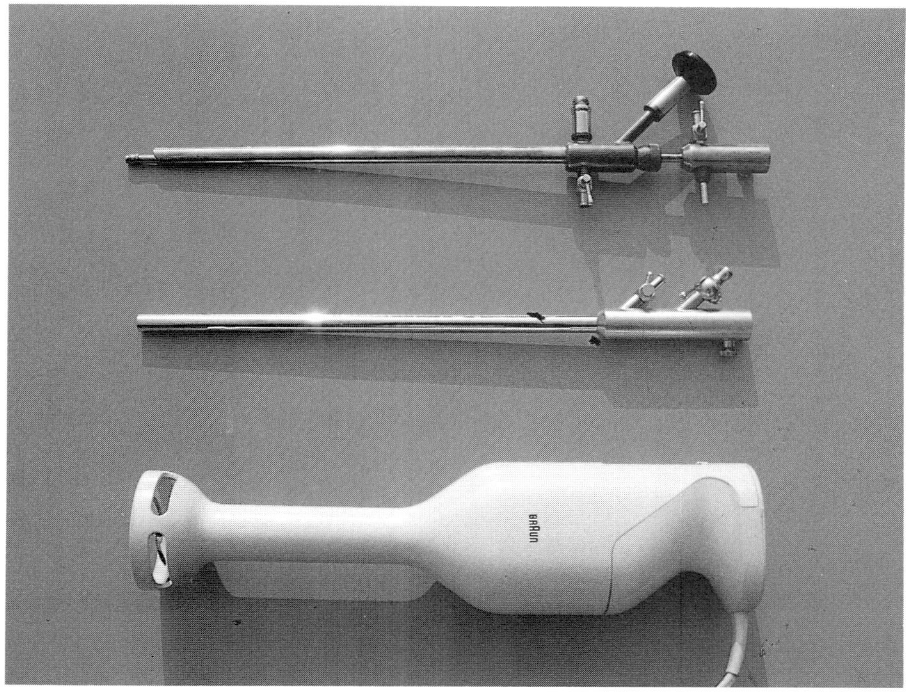

Fig. 3.22 The endoscopic liquidizer and surgical aspirator (middle). It has been used to morcellate nephrectomy specimens within the retrieval bag but, like many of its counterparts, is often obstructed by fibrous tissue components. The principle, based on a kitchen blender (bottom), has also been used for a 5 mm endoscopic device for the prostate (top).

too bulky to bring out directly through the abdominal wall. Impermeability to all cells is also essential.

Once the neck of the retrieval bag has been brought out to the surface, then any further dissection or morcellation becomes extracorporeal and there is no danger of seeding possible tumour cells back into the peritoneum.

Morcellating devices

Morcellating devices are required when the tissue bulk is greater than the diameter of the port. There are a variety of crude devices available at the moment, and we are certain to see a great refinement of these in the near future. At present, the main problem is the morcellation and removal of fibrous connective tissue, which causes the instrument to malfunction. At present, there is not very much difference between inserting a pair of blunt-nosed Mayo scissors and fragmenting the tissue and the electrical devices which either liquidize or morcellate the tissue (Fig. 3.22).

One of the disadvantages of removing tissue in a liquidized or morcellated state is that accurate staging of a possible tumour by the histopathologist is very difficult, if not sometimes impossible. This means that preoperative staging must be as thorough as possible and in the case of renal tumours, a CT scan is essential in every case when previously one might have operated solely with an IVU and ultrasound. However, the type of tissue and possible tumour can easily be identified even with liquidized samples.

References

KeyMed (1992) Optical tests for comparison of laparoscopes/video systems. KeyMed (Medical and Industrial Equipment) Ltd.

O'Boyle P. (1990) Videoendoscopy. The remote operating technique. *British Journal of Urology*, **65**, 557–9.

4: General Laparoscopic Techniques

M.J. COPTCOAT AND A.D. JOYCE

Introduction

The peritoneum is the largest and most complex serous membrane in the body. The part lining the abdominal wall (parietes) is called the parietal peritoneum, whilst that lining the viscera is the visceral peritoneum. The parietal and visceral layers are in actual contact and are lubricated by a small quantity of serous fluid which allows them to glide over each other. The insufflating gas is injected into the potential space between the two layers, called the peritoneal cavity.

The parietal peritoneum is only loosely applied to the abdominal wall anteriorly, where it derives its blood supply and innervation. Since these nerves carry sensory information in A delta somatic fibres to the dorsal columns of the spinal cord, injury or irritation of the parietal peritoneum produces acute or 'sharp' pain. It can be abolished with local anaesthesia for insertion of trocars but although this is adequate for diagnostic laparoscopy, muscle paralysis is essential for free manipulation of multiple instruments which in turn necessitates a general anaesthetic with ventilation. Assisted ventilation is also useful in artificially reversing the acidosis that can occur from prolonged carbon dioxide absorption. Thus you have the apparent anomaly of a day-case minimally invasive procedure that requires paralysis and assisted ventilation.

On the other hand, the visceral peritoneum is very closely applied to the viscera it invests and from which it receives its blood supply and innervation. These nerves carry sensory information in C fibres of the sympathetic nervous system and do not cause pain in response to direct injury such as burning or clipping but rather to stretching and distension which is minimal during laparoscopic procedures.

Laparoscopic inspection of the peritoneal cavity requires identification and opening up of the potential space between the visceral and parietal peritoneal layers. The space can be difficult to find, especially in the obese and in patients who have undergone previous intra-abdominal surgery with subsequent adhesion formation. Early pioneers placed their first port through a minilaparotomy, but with the advent of the safe Veress needle, a simple and safe technique can be quickly mastered for the majority of patients and a minilaparotomy reserved for those with adhesions.

Once the needle is in the correct compartment, flow of gas must be sufficient to maintain an adequate space for inspection and surgery. Following the introduction of the gas into the peritoneal cavity, the intracavity pressure rises to a level which depends on the volume of gas and the compliance of the cavity. Lower pressures are necessary to achieve good visualization when the abdominal wall is completely relaxed and the passively distended abdomen forms a marquee in which the surgery is performed with an audience. Pressures of 10 cmH_2O are usually deemed adequate. Higher pressures may exceed capillary pressure and prevent absorption of gas into the portal and systemic circulation but locally produce unwanted congestion and difficult haemostasis.

Operating theatre layout

Operative laparoscopy is high technology, and whilst the urologist should be familiar with all of his or her equipment, there is no doubt that the success of complicated laparoscopic procedures depends on the whole team. Nursing staff and technicians may need to receive specialized training in the care and maintenance of new equipment. Simple advice, such as avoiding pointed towel clips when stabilizing camera and light leads, is vital to prevent damage but is not usually part of the standard operating nurse training.

The position of the patient, operator and assistant has been described for each separate technique in this book. The monitors should always be placed directly opposite the operator and assistant. A slave monitor for the assistant is ergonomically much more satisfactory. Racked systems which include light source, insufflator, camera unit and video recorder occupy less space but it is important always to keep the diathermy machine as far away from the imaging system as possible to reduce diathermy interference. The ideal position for the scrub nurse will vary for each surgeon especially if this nurse is also acting as an assistant. The scrub nurse must also have easy access to a laparotomy set, which must always be available. It will seldom be used, but when it is required, it will probably be for an emergency.

Despite all of these extra lessons that need to be learned by both urologists and nurses alike, these are exciting times to be involved in operative laparoscopy. The principles have become established and the opportunity is there for all to contribute in refining our techniques and sharing universally in a surgical subspecialty that is rewarding to participate in, fun to watch and is definitely the way ahead.

Formation of a pneumoperitoneum

The common starting point for all laparoscopic procedures is the formation of a pneumoperitoneum. The initial puncturing needle through which gas is insufflated has traditionally been called a Veress

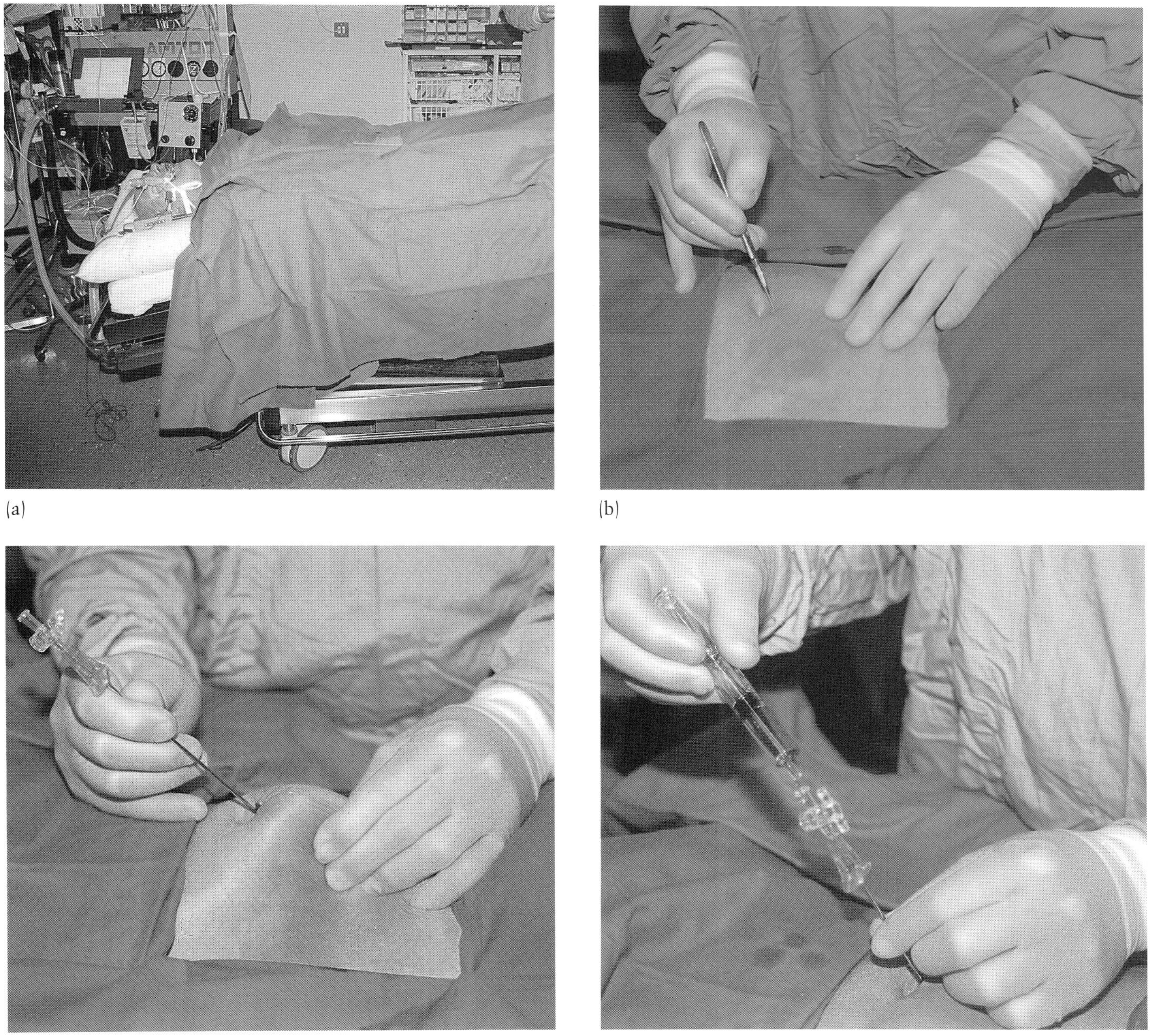

(a) (b) (c) (d)

Fig. 4.1 Preparations for creating a pneumoperitoneum for pelvic laparoscopy. (a) The patient is prepared in a 25% head-down position. (b) A hemicircular incision is made below the umbilicus. (c) The Veress needle is inserted at 45° into the pelvis, whilst the abdomen wall is lifted. (d) The needle position is checked with the drop test (see main text).

needle. This is also available as a disposable needle with the same safety mechanism as the trocars and cannulae. The needle is held as a dart and pushed into the abdominal space, helped by the pulling up of a fold of the abdomen (Fig. 4.1c). There are three quick tests that strongly suggest that the needle has been satisfactorily positioned. First, aspirate. Secondly, infuse 3–5 ml of saline. There should be no resistance. Finally, witness a drop of saline receding down the needle because of the relative vacuum created by lifting up the abdominal wall (Fig. 4.1d). These tests have a small false negative rate and it is interesting that our gynaecological colleagues rarely use them. The

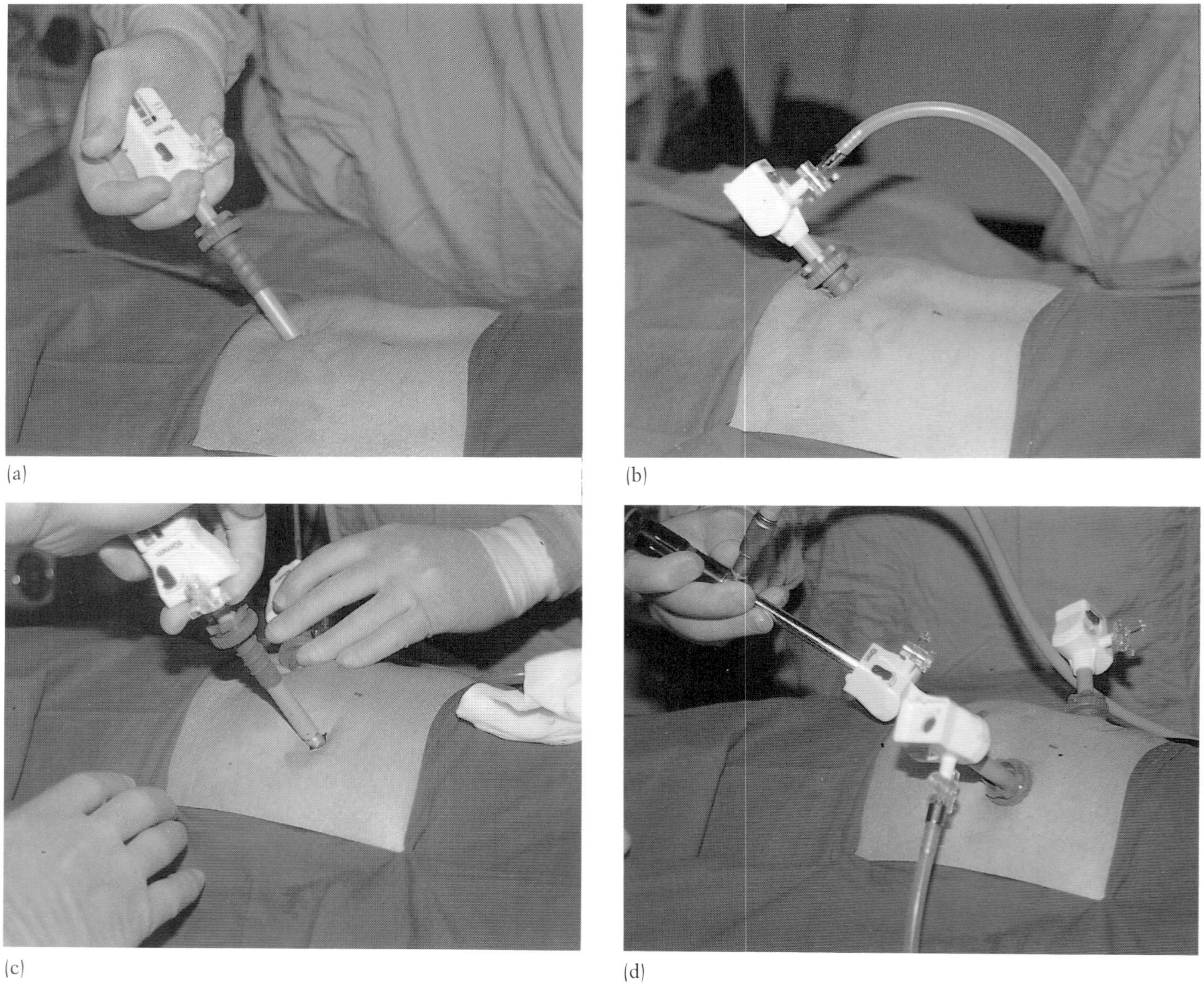

Fig. 4.2 Placement the telescope port and secondary ports. (a) A 10mm disposable port is inserted below the umbilicus for the telescope. (b) Carbon dioxide is initially transferred to the telescope port. (c) Secondary ports are inserted. (d) Carbon dioxide is connected to a secondary port to prevent cooling of the telescope.

needle is then connected to a gas insufflator. Modern insufflators not only provide varying flow rates and a measure of the volume and pressure infused but can also be set to an automatic mode which is invaluable during long procedures. If the initial infusion pressure is above 10mm of mercury then one must suspect that the Veress needle is not lying free within the abdomen or is trapped in omentum or behind bowel. This can usually be corrected by simple repositioning of the tip. Subsequent pressures again should not exceed 10mm of mercury because it is felt that this would severely impede the venous return through intra-abdominal organs over a period of several hours and increase the splinting effect on the diaphragm. However, this is very much a theoretical concept, and work still needs to be done concerning the possible hazards of very long laparoscopic procedures. Up until now, we have, perhaps naively, felt that the anaesthetic risks of

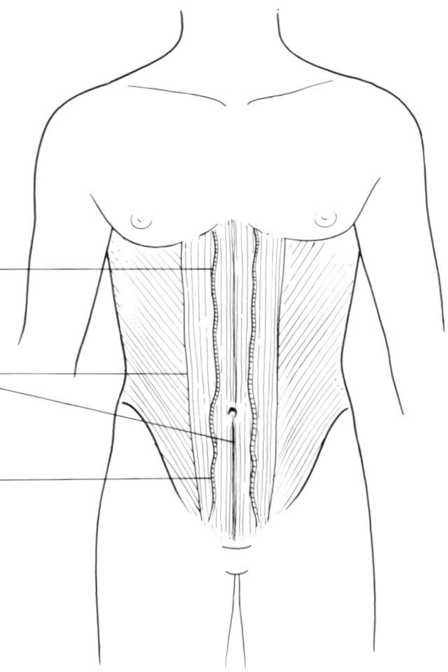

Fig. 4.3 The inferior epigastric artery coursing along the rectus sheath, anastomosing with the superior epigastric artery, is the source of frustrating complications of secondary port placement. The ideal port sites are in the midline or at the edge of the rectus sheath in the semilunar line.

a long laparoscopic nephrectomy were similar to the transatlantic crossing by a jumbo jet where the only dangers are concerned with the very beginning and end of the procedure.

Port placement

A 10 or 12mm trocar and cannula is then inserted into the abdomen for initial laparoscopic viewing (Fig. 4.2a). This is traditionally done through a small skin incision on the periphery of the umbilicus. This site has mainly been used for its cosmetic advantages and we are now finding that there are many instances when the camera should be placed elsewhere.

One golden rule to follow is that the viewing laparoscope, with or without its associated camera, should be inserted away from the site of operation. This provides the potential for both close-up and distant wide-angle views once several instruments are in the operative field. The sites of the midline and semilunar lines are chosen because of the absence of muscle at these potential points of entry and both are guaranteed to miss the superficial epigastric vessels which run up through the rectus muscles (Fig. 4.3). Subsequent ports should always be sited after internal illumination with the house lights off. This shows that one is clear of abdominal wall vessels. A transverse skin incision is made which will form a snug fit around the cannula and grip. The ports should be inserted under direct endoscopic vision and removal of ports should also be visualized in case a vessel had been perforated that will haemorrhage postoperatively without the tamponading effect of the cannula. Grips that hold the port firmly in the muscle fascia are preferred because one can safely withdraw all but

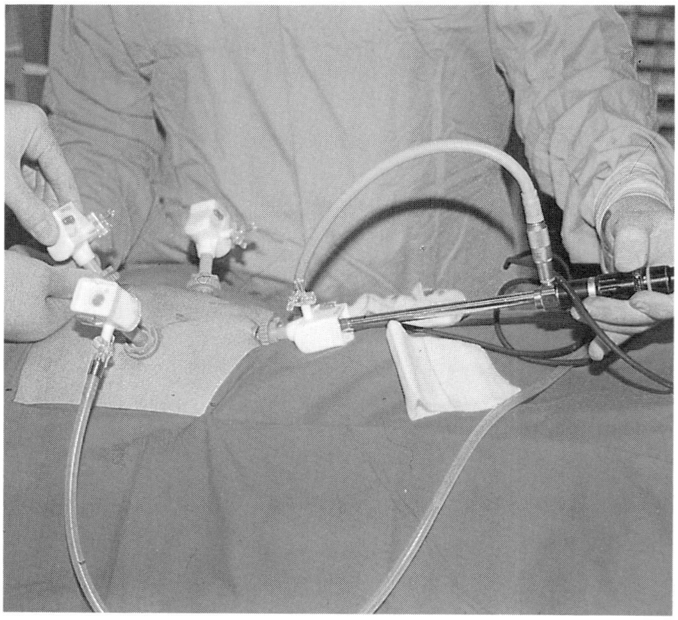

Fig. 4.4 The position of the telescope port grip is checked by looking retrogradely from a secondary port.

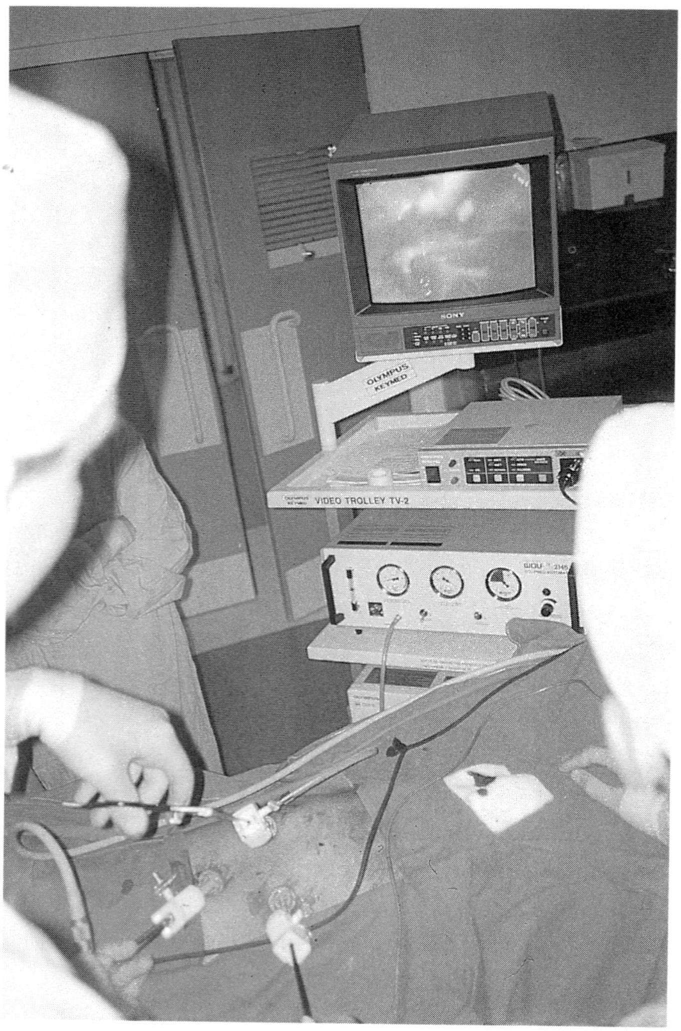

Fig. 4.5 With the pneumoperitoneum achieved, and all the ports in place, operative video laparoscopy can begin.

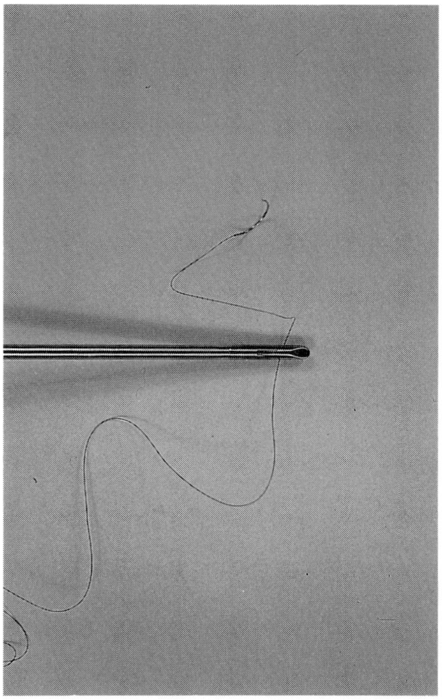

Fig. 4.6 The laparoscopic suture should be grasped 3–4 cm proximal to the needle. Then even a curved needle can be pulled through a port if the valve is momentarily depressed.

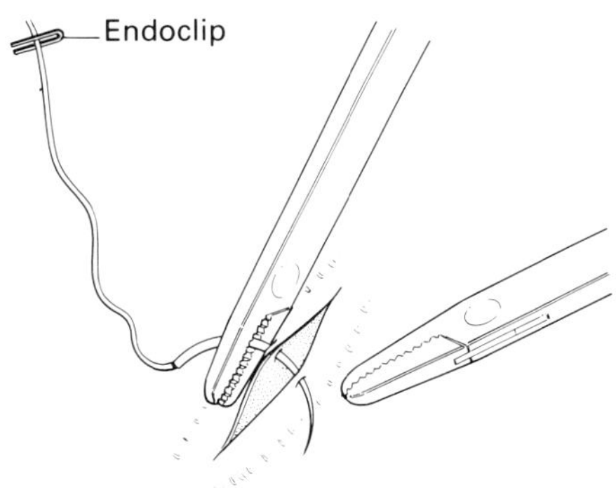

Fig. 4.7 A quick technique to start a continuous suture is to place a clip at the opposite end of the suture material to the needle. This technique can also be used to complete a continuous suture. The clip is less likely to slide off from braided sutures.

1 cm of the port from the abdomen. This produces a greater range for forceps to open and allows the telescope to provide a very wide field of view when required.

Laparoscopic suturing techniques

Laparoscopic suturing is a difficult technique, and at the present time there is little need for it in urological laparoscopy. However, unexpected situations may be encountered such as an omental tear or bowel perforation during a difficult trocar insertion. Having been presented with a patient requiring a nephrectomy who had undergone three previous major abdominal operations, Coptcoat found the pneumoperitoneum to be straightforward but insertion of the first trocar very difficult. Adhesions held the transverse colon close to the abdominal wall and a perforation was made with this trocar. This was recognized during initial inspection when he found that he was viewing the inside of the large bowel rather than the peritoneal cavity. Insertion of two ports adjacent to this area allowed him to inspect the iatrogenic bowel perforation. The perforation could be oversewn with two layers of interrupted sutures using an intracorporeal technique. The transperitoneal laparoscopic nephrectomy could then go ahead as planned. Such a complication and its remedy using suturing techniques is unusual but the example provides evidence of the capabilities of such suturing techniques.

What we will undoubtedly see is an expansion of urological laparoscopy in which suture anastomoses will be the first choice until stapling anastomotic techniques are refined both in terms of instrumentation and the application of absorbable staples. At the present time, a laparoscopic pyeloplasty is best done with a continuous intracorporeal laparoscopic suture.

Generally speaking, special laparoscopic needles and sutures are not required. Most straight needles and some curved needles can easily be introduced through 10 mm ports. The suture material should be grasped with a pair of forceps approximately 3–4 cm proximal to the needle itself and the needle then dragged through the port. The flap valve, if present, should be depressed momentarily during this manoeuvre (Fig. 4.6).

Continuous suture

The suture line is cut to the desired length. Excess suture material is difficult to handle intracorporeally. The traditional method of tying a knot at the beginning and end of the continuous suture can be reproduced within the abdomen but is tedious and time-consuming. A far quicker technique is to place a clip at the opposite end of the suture material to the needle; this is firmly tightened (Fig. 4.7). A continuous

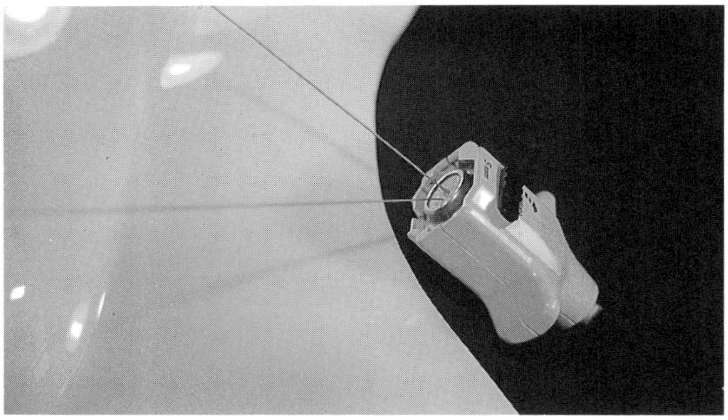
(a)

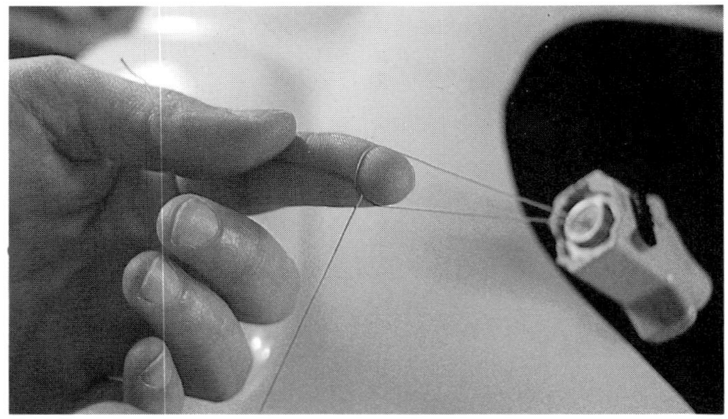
(b)

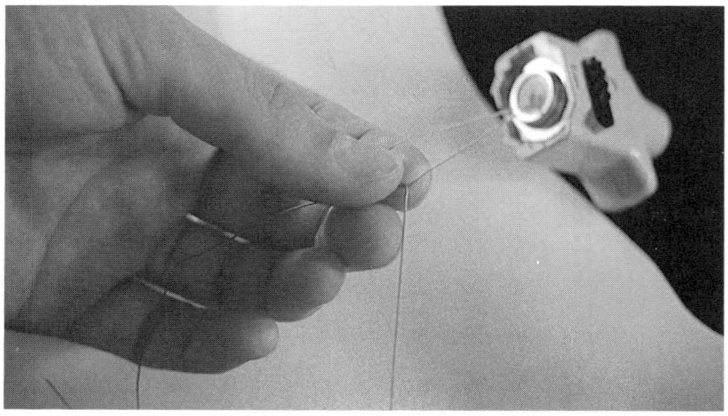
(c)

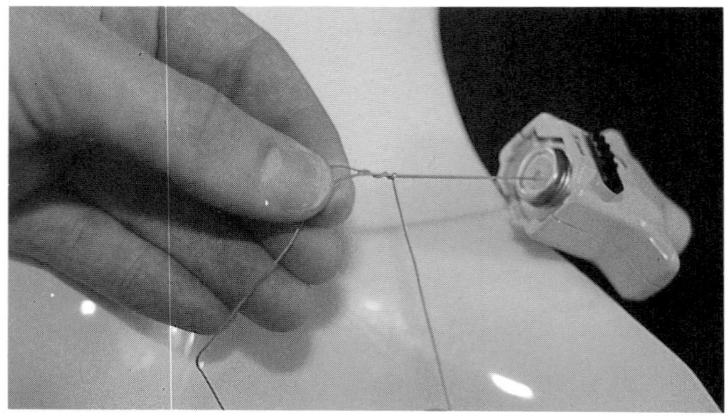
(d)

Fig. 4.8 The extracorporeal knot technique. (a) The two ends are withdrawn through the port. (b) A single throw knot is made. (c) The throw knot is held with thumb and second finger. (d) Three revolutions are made around both strands. (e) This knot is recommended when using monofilament suture materials. (f) The lust is pushed down with a knot tier. (g) The suture is then finished and cut.

suture is made using an endoscopic needle-holder and a grasper. The function of the grasping forceps is to present the needle in the right position in relation to the needle-holder, to grasp the needle when it is passed through the tissue and to control the tension on the suture as it is drawn through the tissue. It also helps to depress the tissue at the anticipated needle exit point should the needle tip be too difficult to see. This provides a better exposure of the needle. A wider field panoramic view is more desirable for suturing because of the relatively wide arc of movements that the instruments follow. When the continuous suture is finished, it is fastened off with a clip and cut. This technique allows for a suture line of only a few centimetres thus making the manipulation easier.

Interrupted suture

Numerous techniques of knot-tying have been described, including intracorporeal and extracorporeal procedures.

The intracorporeal technique requires intensive training and practice but has few indications in urological laparoscopy. It is possible to tie almost all of the sutures outside of the abdomen. The needle is introduced into the abdomen. The opposite end can be secured outside with small forceps to avoid its accidentally sliding into the

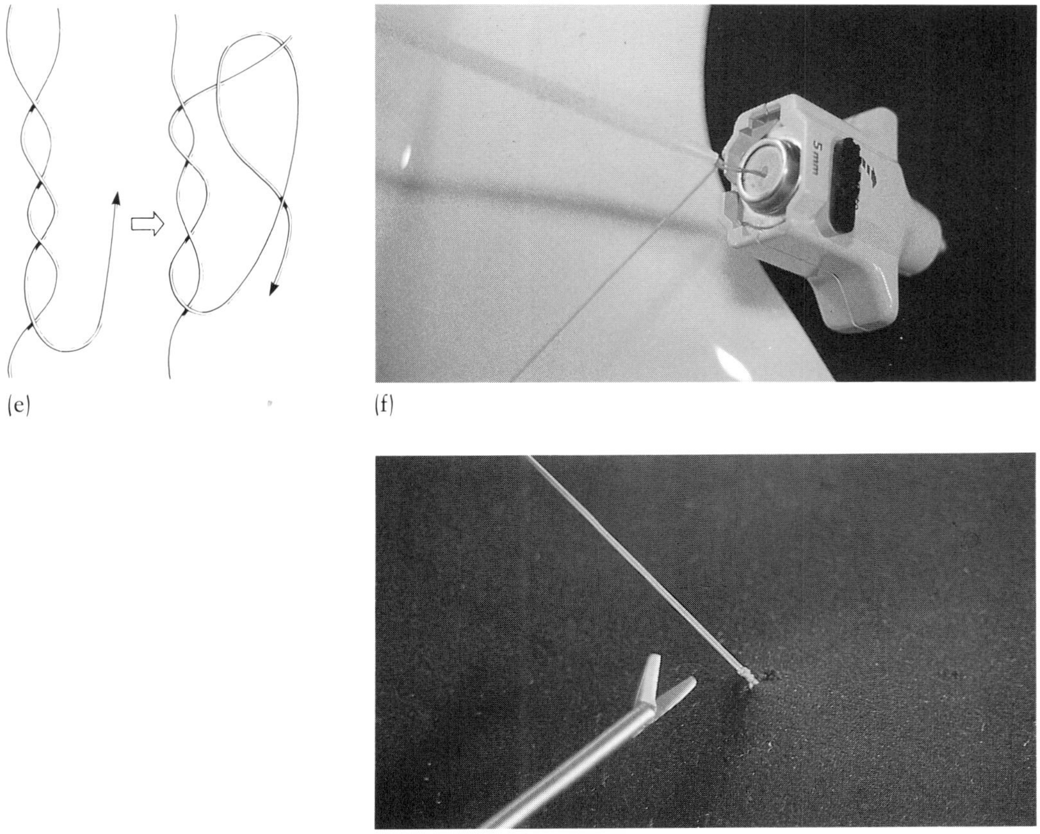

Fig. 4.8 *Contd*

(e) (f) (g)

operative field. The needle is passed through the tissue as previously described and then withdrawn through that same port. A single throw knot is made with the two suture ends. This knot is held with the thumb and second finger. With the free end of the suture, three revolutions are made around both suture strands. The tail of the suture is inserted through the first loop and then though the loop that was formed below the initial single throw knot. This is a fisherman's knot (Fig. 4.8). The tail is pulled up and cut. By simply pulling the end of the thread, the knot slides down by itself. It is then pushed with a knot tier or atraumatic forceps and secured. Finally, the suture is cut off 3mm from the knot.

Intracorporeal knot-tying is merely a reproduction of those techniques we use at open surgery. The movements are more difficult when restricted to laparoscopic instruments and their angle of entry, but with practice and, in particular, with shorter lengths of suture material, such intracorporeal suturing can be mastered (Fig. 4.9).

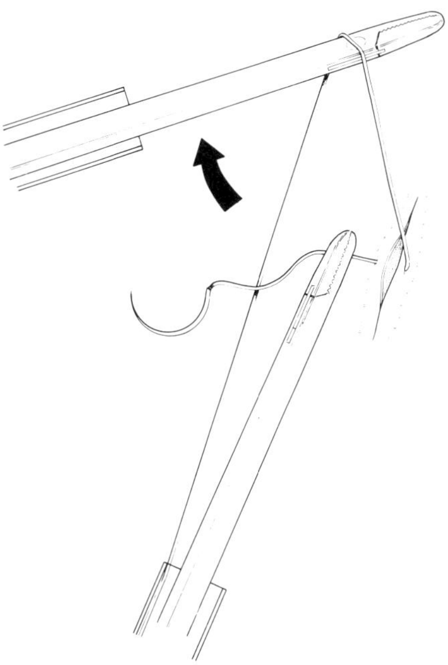

Fig. 4.9 Intracorporeal knot-tying is time-consuming, but the point of manipulation is close to the point tissue approximation, and so tears are less likely.

Wound closures

The use of larger ports (e.g. 10, 12 and 16mm) has made the possibility of a postoperative wound hernia more likely. In these instances, the wound should be closed at the end of the operation by placing a

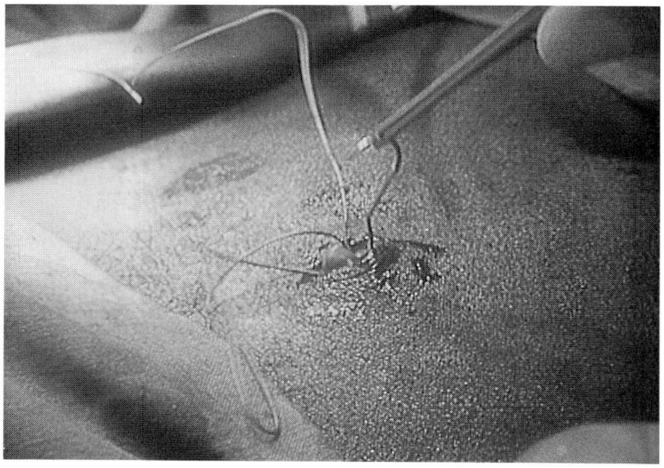

Fig. 4.10 Port wounds of 10mm or more should receive a fascial suture to prevent wound-herniation.

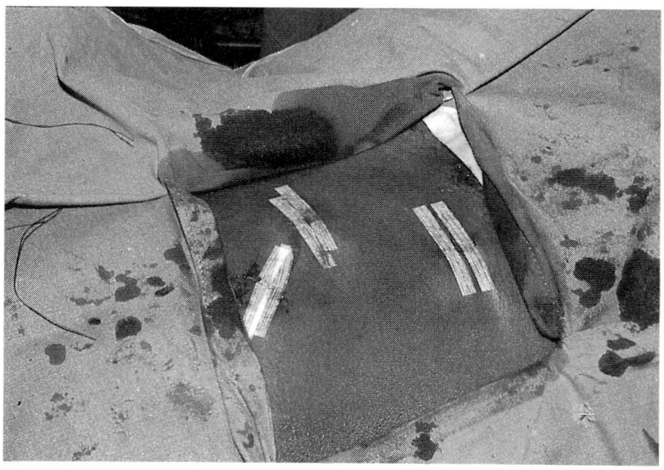

Fig. 4.11 Skin wounds can be closed with a subcuticular suture, or as in this case, with steristrips. The cosmetic result is excellent.

suture across the fascia (Fig. 4.10). If there is any difficulty in picking up the fascia externally, a large hand needle can be passed through with endoscopic guidance from below. The skin can then be closed separately either with a subcuticular suture or a steristrip (Fig. 4.11). Dexon seems to produce a slight hypertrophy of the scar which can mar the external appearance of a successful minimally invasive procedure. Something nonabsorbable is to be preferred.

5: Anaesthesia for Laparoscopy

D. GREEN AND A. MITCHELL

Introduction

Following the introduction of gynaecological laparoscopy doubts were soon expressed about the difficulties and dangers inherent in a seemingly simple and relatively noninvasive technique. As a result of investigations into the effects of peritoneal insufflation of carbon dioxide during laparoscopy, Hodgson *et al.* (1970) concluded, 'Though laparoscopy offers advantages to both patients and surgeon it involves considerable alteration in respiratory and cardiovascular homeostasis and should not be regarded as yet another minor investigation.' However, it is only with the recent introduction of more prolonged techniques, such as laparoscopic nephrectomy, that the full scale of these 'alterations' has manifested itself. Both the anaesthetist and the surgeon must be aware of the pathophysiological effects of laparoscopy so that the patient can receive optimum benefit from the technique and experience minimum complications.

Anaesthetic techniques

General anaesthetic techniques for laparoscopy do not differ markedly from those used for other surgical procedures. However, in recent years the spectrum of laparoscopic techniques has widened from simple laparoscopic sterilization in gynaecology lasting a few minutes to the more complex urological procedures, such as laparoscopic nephrectomy, which may take up to seven hours. For ambulatory procedures, opioid supplementation should be minimized as this may delay recovery and increase the risk of postoperative nausea and vomiting .

Is endotracheal intubation mandatory?

A long-standing debate regarding the necessity for endotracheal intubation (ETI) during the shorter gynaecological laparoscopic procedures has continued for the last 20 years. Since the majority of these procedures are carried out in day-surgery units, reducing the incidence of sore throat from ETI or muscle pains associated with the relaxant suxamethonium is seen as a major advantage of avoiding ETI (Kenefick *et al.* 1987).

Nevertheless, during longer procedures, the combination of a head-down tilt and pneumoperitoneum could increase the risk of regurgitation of gastric contents, especially in the obese patient. In these cases, ETI is employed.

Is mechanical ventilation mandatory?

Hypoventilation in the spontaneously breathing patient is exacerbated by a head-down tilt and diaphragmatic splinting from the pneumoperitoneum. This, together with carbon dioxide absorption (if carbon dioxide is used as the insufflating gas) leads to hypercapnea. The association of ventricular dysrhythmias, hypercapnea and halothane anaesthesia thus led to a preference for mechanical ventilation to control $PaCO_2$ during gynaecological laparoscopy (Hodgson *et al.* 1970). Although newer inhalational agents, such as isoflurane, are much less likely to cause dysrhythmias in the spontaneously breathing patient undergoing laparoscopy for shorter procedures (Kenefick *et al.* 1987), longer cases make mechanical ventilation mandatory, as carbon dioxide absorption may be considerable (Blobner *et al.* 1992).

Is muscle paralysis mandatory?

Having decided to intubate and ventilate the patient, is it necessary to maintain neuromuscular blockade throughout the procedure? During complex intra-abdominal surgery such as nephrectomy, visualization depends on adequate separation of the visceral and parietal layers of the peritoneum, and this can only be achieved by complete relaxation (high compliance) of the abdominal wall musculature, if high intra-abdominal pressures are to be avoided.

In addition, avoidance of sudden patient movement (e.g. coughing) is necessary to prevent inadvertent injury. In these cases, muscle paralysis must be sustained throughout the procedure, and the effects of the neuromuscular blocker must be monitored with a peripheral nerve stimulator.

Is nitrous oxide contraindicated?

Concerns have been expressed over the use of nitrous oxide during prolonged laparoscopic surgery because of its puted ability to cause bowel distension which might hinder surgical access (Eger & Saidman 1965, Marco *et al.* 1990) and a puted increased risk of postoperative nausea and vomiting (PONV). The latter is highly relevant if the patient is being treated as a day case as it may delay discharge from the unit or even require overnight admission if protracted. Recent work has demonstrated no deleterious effects of nitrous oxide on bowel distension during laparoscopic cholecystectomy (Taylor *et al.* 1992) and the effects on PONV have been vigorously disputed in the anaesthetic literature (Watcha & White 1992, Hartung 1993).

Fluid replacement

Hypotension is a frequent accompaniment to laparoscopy, especially if performed in the head-up position, and occurs more commonly during laparoscopic than during conventional cholecystectomy (Rose *et al.* 1992). Adequate fluid replacement reduces the incidence of hypotension (Fishburne & Keith 1977).

During laparoscopy, blood loss is difficult to assess, as only a small area of the surgical field is visible at any time. Classical signs of occult bleeding such as hypotension, tachycardia and reduction in urine output (if measured) are unreliable during anaesthesia. A high index of suspicion and frequent inspection of the peritoneal cavity by the surgeon are necessary if bleeding is suspected and appropriate volume replacement instituted.

Monitoring

Cardiography

ECG monitoring is mandatory during any procedure under general anaesthesia. Dysrhythmias are particularly common during laparoscopy, primarily because of the effects of hypercarbia and associated catecholamine secretion potentiating the effects of halothane on the heart. The introduction of neuromuscular blocking drugs with little vagolytic action, (e.g. atracurium and vecuronium) together with potent opioids (e.g. fentanyl) increase the likelihood of bradycardia during laparoscopy.

Noninvasive blood pressure (NIBP)

Pneumoperitoneum and head-up tilt (as during laparoscopic cholecystectomy) reduce cardiac performance, so a fall in blood pressure must be anticipated (Rose *et al.* 1992, Noirot *et al.* 1992). Other causes of cardiovascular collapse and hypotension are noted in the section on haemodynamics. Automatic NIBP measurements must be made at frequent intervals (5 minutes or less).

Pulse oximetry

Hypoxaemia is a common accompaniment to laparoscopy due to pre-existing lung pathology, equipment failure and poor anaesthetic technique (e.g. oesophageal or endobronchial intubation), hypoventilation, intrapulmonary shunting and reduced cardiac output (Cunningham & Schlanger 1992). Continuous monitoring of arterial oxygen saturation is mandatory at all times, from induction of anaesthesia until full patient recovery has occurred.

Capnography

End-tidal monitoring of carbon dioxide tension is necessary for determining optimum ventilation rate and depth for the patient who is mechanically ventilated. It is closely related to arterial carbon dioxide tensions during laparoscopy (McKinstry *et al.* 1992). Simple calculation of minute volume from standard charts is inadequate during prolonged insufflation of carbon dioxide, as absorption of gas through the peritoneum adds significantly to carbon dioxide levels in the blood in some patients. In patients who are allowed to breathe spontaneously, a raised end-tidal carbon dioxide tension suggests the need to ventilate.

Temperature

During procedures lasting more than one hour (e.g. lymphadenectomy and nephrectomy), naso-pharyngeal temperature must be monitored. Rectal temperature may not give an accurate representation of core temperature during pneumoperitoneum. Body temperature falls after induction of anaesthesia, as warmer core blood distributes to the cooler periphery. This is due to inhibition of neurones in the preoptic hypothalamic nuclei (POH) which also control the body's response to thermal stress. General anaesthetics such as halothane, together with opioids such as fentanyl, depress the threshold for vasoconstriction under anaesthesia by 2–3°C.

By promoting peripheral vasodilation, inhalational anaesthetics increase heat loss by radiation, conduction and evaporation. The use of neuromuscular blockers inhibits heat production by abolition of shivering (Green 1993). Active measures must be taken to maintain body heat, such as humidification of inspired gases, warming blankets, keeping the operating theatre warm (21–23°C) and warming all fluids given intravenously. Previous anecdotal evidence suggested that the cold insufflating gas also contributed to reducing patient temperature. However, our studies using intra-abdominal thermistors during laparoscopic procedures have shown that the intra-abdominal temperature only fluctuates close to the CO_2 entry port and that over 5 cm away the temperature is maintained within 1°C despite flows of up to 700 l of CO_2 (M.J. Coptcoat & M. Matuszewski, personal communication).

Invasive monitoring of central venous and arterial pressure

Invasive monitoring of central venous and arterial pressure is desirable for those procedures, such as laparoscopic nephrectomy and cystectomy, where blood loss rarely but realistically can be considerable and there is a delay in even immediate open exploration.

Patient position

Great care should be taken to ensure the patient pressure points are well padded during prolonged procedures to prevent skin and nerve ischaemia. In addition, the steep head-down tilt sometimes necessary for bowel displacement during lymphadenectomy requires that a non-slip mattress be used on the operating table.

Insufflating gases

The insufflating gas must be:
nonirritant
nonflammable (as diathermy is frequently used)
soluble in blood (to minimize the effects of inadvertent intravascular injection)
cost-effective.

Although air was used initially, it is 20 times less soluble than carbon dioxide, so the results of inadvertent intravascular injection would be catastrophic. It also supports combustion.

Nitrous oxide has been advocated by some as it is nearly as soluble as carbon dioxide, it does not impose a CO_2 load (Corrall *et al.* 1974) and causes less peritoneal irritation (Uhlich 1982). However, it can form explosive mixtures in combination with methane gas escaping through the bowel wall, so its use has been abandoned in those cases where a diathermy must be used. Nevertheless, it remains popular for diagnostic procedures carried out under local anaesthetic (Uhlich 1982).

Carbon dioxide has been found, overall, to be the most satisfactory gas for insufflation. Doubts have been expressed concerning the extent of CO_2 absorption from the peritoneal cavity. Seed *et al.* (1970) did not find it a problem in patients who were mechanically ventilated and considered the amount absorbed to be small. Nevertheless, Hodgson *et al.* (1970) found it sufficiently large to recommend mechanical ventilation in patients undergoing laparoscopy. By measurement of both oxygen uptake and carbon dioxide production using a metabolic computer, Blobner *et al.* (1992) have confirmed an increase in carbon dioxide uptake during laparoscopic cholecystectomy. In one case, the accidental production of subcutaneous CO_2 emphysema resulted in a marked increase in $V\text{CO}_2$ and a raised $Pa\text{CO}_2$ despite an increase in minute ventilation to 200 ml kg^{-1} min^{-1}. Blobner *et al.* also confirmed that higher intra-abdominal pressures protect against further absorption of gas by compressing the venous capillaries of the peritoneum.

The reason for these different results is due to the fact that carbon dioxide absorption from the peritoneum is a complex interaction between:

volume and tension of gas insufflated
solubility of the gas in blood
escape into the tissue (causing emphysema)
perfusion of the cavity walls (and the consequent ability of the venous drainage to transport the gas into the portal or systemic circulation).

Given the variation in amount of gas insufflated, intracavity pressure and venous drainage, it is not surprising that differences have been found in CO_2 uptake. As far as inadvertent CO_2 embolism is concerned, it is reassuring to note that radiologists have rapidly injected 50–100ml of carbon dioxide for cardiac contrast studies with no ill effects (Lewis *et al.* 1972). Up to 7.5$ml\,kg^{-1}$ of CO_2 has been tolerated intravenously whereas only 0.25$ml\,kg^{-1}$ has proven lethal in cats (Yacoub *et al.* 1982). The rapidity with which CO_2 is excreted by the lungs and absorbed into the body stores makes it the safest gas at present in use.

Pathophysiological effects of laparoscopy

Haemodynamic

The haemodynamic effects of laparoscopy extend from minor hypotensive episodes requiring no specific treatment to cardiac arrest. They are the result of a complex interaction between the following:

- Patient position can cause a decrease in venous return, being particularly noted where a pronounced head-up tilt is used. In addition to general anaesthesia and mechanical ventilation, this can result in a marked reduction in cardiac output, although blood pressure is usually maintained by an increase in systemic vascular resistance (Noirot *et al.* 1992).
- Hypoventilation because of a head-down position or absorption of carbon dioxide leads to hypercarbia which can induce dysrhythmias and a fall in cardiac output (Fishburne & Keith 1977).
- Blood loss, as in any surgical procedure, causes reduced venous return and reduced cardiac output.
- Perforation of a major vessel or viscus by a trocar can occur prior to insertion of the laparoscope and may go unnoticed initially.
- Traction or stimulation of visceral peritoneum may induce a vasovagal response, resulting in bradycardia and even cardiac arrest (Fishburne & Keith 1977). This can be prevented by the use of vagolytic drugs, such as atropine.

Gas embolus is one of the most feared complications of laparoscopy but it is fortunately an extremely rare complication (Phillips *et al.* 1976). Signs of gas embolus include hypotension, cardiac dysrhythmias, a fall in oxygen saturation and cardiac arrest. The presence of a 'mill wheel' murmur over the precordium is suggestive, but the only absolute criterion is the presence of gas in the circulation. Differential diagnosis of cardiac collapse includes any of the above causes, but if gas embolus is suspected urgent measures must be taken.

Since cardiac output is impeded by the compressible pocket of gas which usually ends up in the right ventricular outflow tract, these measures include immediate cessation of insufflation, turning the patient on the left side in a slight head-down position and aspiration of air from the right ventricle following insertion of a central venous catheter (Yacoub *et al.* 1982). The latter should not be necessary with carbon dioxide as the insufflating gas as it is rapidly absorbed into the blood stream.

It is sensible to administer 100% oxygen during this time as hypoxaemia is certain to be an accompaniment. If the gas enters visceral veins then air may be trapped in the portal circulation and this can result in delayed death from gas embolism.

Is laparoscopy safer for the cardiac or haemodynamically compromised patient than an equivalent open procedure? Few studies have directly addressed this aspect although a recent examination of the cardiovascular changes associated with a raised intra-abdominal pressure (due to insufflation) concluded that the 'haemodynamic changes produced could be deleterious in patients with compromised cardiac function' (Noirot *et al.* 1992).

Hypotension was found to be a 'common problem' during laparoscopic cholecystectomy versus open in a retrospective case note study (Rose *et al.* 1992).

Respiratory

Hypercapnoea

Many early studies concentrated on the adverse effects of patient position (head-down) and raised IAP causing a reduction in minute volume. This led to recommendations to ventilate the patient (Seed *et al.*, Hodgson *et al.* 1970). During shorter procedures in slim patients, spontaneous ventilation using a face mask is acceptable and does not lead to significant hypercarbia, acidosis or cardiac arrhythmias (Kenefick *et al.* 1987).

Diaphragmatic function is compromised both by raised IAP and the full weight of the viscera being borne by the diaphragm in the head-down position. In addition, the fall in functional residual capacity causes an increased shunt and subsequent hypoxaemia (Fishburne & Keith 1977).

Absorption of gases, particularly carbon dioxide, may lead to hypoxaemia and hypercapnoea as stated earlier, continuing after cessation of insufflation and even into the early postoperative period (Lewis *et al.* 1972).

Hypoxaemia

The differential diagnosis of hypoxaemia during laparoscopy includes pre-existing conditions such as respiratory disease, hypoventilation, increased shunting due to such conditions as endobronchial intubation, pneumothorax, subcutaneous emphysema and aspiration of gastric contents, and reduced cardiac output. During laparoscopy, some or all of these factors may be sufficiently severe to preclude adequate oxygenation (i.e. maintenance of oxygen saturation above 90%) and to force abandonment in favour of an open procedure when oxygenation is immediately restored to normal (Cunningham & Schlanger 1992).

Pneumothorax

Pneumothorax may occur during any surgical procedure; that specifically due to laparoscopy may occur as a result of defects in the embryological development of the diaphragm.

The posterior, lateral and central portions are formed by the fusion of the dorsal mesentery and mesoderm with the pleuroperitoneal membrane. This membrane is derived from the pulmonary ridge, so if the mesoderm is not properly deposited at any of these adjacent points of union, a failure of proper fusion may result in congenital diaphragmatic defects.

Increased IAP from insufflation could force gas from the peritoneal to the pleural space. The higher IAP needs to be, in order to produce an adequate pneumoperitoneum, the greater the likelihood of significant pneumothorax in susceptible patients. Reduction of IAP is best achieved by full relaxation of the abdominal wall with specific neuromuscular blocking drugs. In addition, using carbon dioxide as the insufflating gas ensures rapid removal of the gas from the pleural cavity (Doctor & Hussain 1973).

Gastrointestinal

It is commonly supposed that laparoscopy increases the likelihood of regurgitation of gastric contents due to a combination of head-down tilt and raised IAP. In fact, the risk may be much smaller than previously thought, as raised IAP may actually *increase* the pressure of the lower oesophageal sphincter and thus limit regurgitation (Jones *et al.* 1989).

A prospective series of 50,048 laparoscopies studied by a working party indicated only one case of aspiration and this occurred at induction of anaesthesia, an incidence of 0.002% (Chamberlain & Carron Brown 1978). This is much less than the 2% incidence reported by Duffy (1979). Roberts & Goodman (1990) used a pH electrode positioned just above the gastro-oesophageal junction and were unable to demonstrate acid reflux in any of the patients studied. (Note that reflux of acid into the lower oesophagus is not synonymous with acid regurgitation into the lungs.) They concluded that endotracheal intubation is not justified on the grounds of airway protection alone but may be required for the other reasons stated above.

Postoperative effects and complications

Pain

Reduction in surgical trauma in laparoscopic versus open procedures should result in a reduction of postoperative pain, lessened requirement for opioids and earlier return to normal activity.

In a retrospective study of 189 major laparoscopic procedures (101 laparoscopic versus 88 conventional cholecystectomies) there was a statistically significant reduction in excessive pain (4% vs. 12%, $P<0.05$) and narcotic requirement (67% vs 94%, $P<0.01$) in the laparoscopic group (Rose *et al.* 1992).

In an effort to reduce the opioid requirement still further, non-steroidal anti-inflammatory drugs (NSAIDs) have been administered along with conventional opioids on demand. Ketorolac is a popular NSAID in this regard, which can be given intravenously at induction of anaesthesia. When used in this way opioid requirements are reduced in the postoperative period (Liu *et al.* 1992). We have found that the routine use of local anaesthesia (bupivicaine 0.5%) in the port wounds almost abolishes any memory of a laparoscopic procedure in our day-case unit.

Myalgias

Vague shoulder-tip pain, neck stiffness and muscle pains, nausea and headache are common accompaniments to laparoscopy (Kenefick *et al.* 1987). Escape of gas from the peritoneal cavity into the pleural cavity with irritation of the visceral pleura is the presumed cause. Although the exact mechanism is unknown, neck pain and stiffness can be reduced by avoiding suxamethonium as the relaxant (Smith *et al.* 1992).

Nausea and vomiting

Nausea and vomiting are common accompaniments to laparoscopy, especially gynaecological. However, it is doubtful whether it is more common following a procedure carried out laparoscopically versus the equivalent open operation. Rose *et al.* (1992) found a similar incidence of nausea and vomiting in patients receiving open versus laparoscopic cholecystectomy. Unfortunately, increased use of NSAIDs in place of opioids has not resulted in a reduction in this unpleasant side-effect (Liu *et al.* 1992).

Respiratory function

Major reductions in peak expiratory flow rate (PEFR), forced expiratory volume in 1 second (FEV_1) and forced vital capacity (FVC) are seen after upper abdominal surgery. It is presumed that replacement of a major (painful) abdominal incision by multiple small ones would produce an improvement in lung function.

This would be particularly appropriate for patients with pre-existing lung pathology who are at high risk of developing upper respiratory tract infection. In a study of 20 patients randomly assigned to laparoscopic or open cholecystectomy, Putensen-Himmer *et al.* (1992) showed that respiratory function is less impaired and recovery improved. For instance, at 24 hours post-surgery FEV_1 in the laparoscopic group was 85% of control versus 54% in the open group.

Minimizing deterioration in postoperative lung function by using laparoscopic versus open cholecystectomy (or nephrectomy) has obvious advantages for patients with pre-existing respiratory dysfunction or those in whom oxygen desaturation *must* be avoided in the post-operative period; for example, patients with sickle cell disease (Davenport *et al.* 1991). However, less convincing differences were seen by Gögler *et al.* (1992) who found a high degree of pulmonary dysfunction in both groups.

Discharge from hospital versus open procedures

No studies have prospectively documented the difference in length of hospital study in laparoscopic versus open procedures, e.g. nephrectomy. Rose *et al.* (1992) looked at hospital outcome in a retrospective comparison and found a significant reduction in hospital stay for laparoscopic (2.5 days) versus open cholecystectomy (6.6. days, $P<0.001$). It would appear that the increased cost of surgical time can be offset by reduced length of hospital stay.

References

Blobner M., Felber A.R., Gögler S., Weigl E.M., Jelen-Esselhorn S. (1992) Carbon dioxide uptake from pneumoperitoneum during laparoscopic cholecystectomy. *Anesthesiology*, **77**, A37.

Chamberlain G.V.P., Carron Brown J.A. eds (1978) Gynaecological laparoscopy: The report of the working party of the confidential enquiry into gynaecological laparoscopy. The Royal College of Obstetricians and Gynaecologists, London.

Corrall I.M., Knights K., Potter D.R., Strunin L. (1974) Arterial oxygen tension during laparoscopy with nitrous oxide in the spontaneously breathing patient. *British Journal of Anaesthesia*, **46**, 925–8.

Cunningham A.J., Schlanger M. (1992) Intraoperative hypoxemia complicating laparoscopic cholecystectomy in a patient with sickle hemoglobinopathy. *Anesthesia Annals*, **75**, 838–43.

Davenport M., Howard E.R., Green D.W. (1991) Minimally invasive surgery in sickle cell disease. *British Medical Journal*, **303**, 249.

Doctor N.H. & Hussain Z. (1973) Bilateral pneumothorax associated with laparoscopy. *Anaesthesia*, **28**, 75–81.

Duffy B.L. (1979) Regurgitation during pelvic laparoscopy. *British Journal of Anaesthesia*, **51**, 1089–90.

Eger E.I. II, Saidman L.J. (1965) Hazards of nitrous oxide anesthesia in bowel obstruction and pneumothorax. *Anesthesiology*, **26**, 61–6.

Fishburne J.I., Keith L. (1977) Anesthesia. In *Laparoscopy* (ed. J.M. Phillips), pp.69–85. Williams and Wilkins, Baltimore.

Gögler S., Felber A.R., Blobner M., Laubrock I., Jelen-Esselhorn S. (1992) Pulmonary function following laparoscopic cholecystectomy versus laparotomic cholecystectomy. *Anesthesiology*, **77**, A10.

Green D.W. (1993) Anaesthesia for microvascular surgery. In *Anaesthesia for Burns, Maxillofacial and Plastic Surgery* (ed. H. Patel), pp.101–2. Edward Arnold, London.

Hartung J. (1993) Nitrous oxide—It's enough to make you vomit. *Anesthesiology*, **78**, 403–5.

Hodgson C., McClelland R.M.A., Newton J.R. (1970) Some effects of the peritoneal insufflation of carbon dioxide at laparoscopy. *Anaesthesia*, **25**, 382–90.

Jones M.J., Mitchell R.W., Hindocha N. (1989) Effect of increased intra-abdominal pressure during laparoscopy on the lower oesophageal sphincter. *Anesthesia Annals*, **68**, 63–5.

Kenefick J.P., Leader A., Maltby J.R., Taylor P.J. (1987) Laparoscopy: blood gas values and minor sequelae associated with three techniques based on isoflurane. *British Journal of Anaesthesia*, **59**, 189–94.

Lewis D.G., Ryder W., Burn N., Wheldon J.T., Tacchi D. (1972) Laparoscopy—an investigation during spontaneous ventilation with halothane. *British Journal of Anaesthesia*, **44**, 685–90.

Liu J., Ding Y., White P.F., Feinstein R., Shear J. (1992) Laparoscopic cholecystectomy: effect of ketorolac on postoperative pain and ventilatory function. *Anesthesiology*, **77**, A1255.

Marco A.P., Yeo C.J., Rock P. (1990) Anesthesia for patients undergoing laparoscopic cholecystectomy. *Anesthesiology*, **73**, 168–170.

McKinstry L.J., Perverseff R.A., Yip R.W. (1992) Arterial and end-tidal carbon dioxide in patients undergoing laparoscopic cholecystectomy. *Anesthesiology*, **77**, A108.

Noirot D., Joris J., Legrand M., Lamy M. (1992) Hemodynamic changes during pneumoperitoneum for laparoscopic cholecystectomy. *Anesthesiology*, **77**, A69.

Phillips J.M., Keith D., Hulka J., Hulka B., Keith L. (1976) Gynecologic laparoscopy in 1975. *Journal of Reproductive Medicine*, **16**, 105-17.

Putensen-Himmer G., Putensen C., Lammer H., Lingnau W., Aigner F., Benzer H. (1992) Comparison of postoperative respiratory function after laparoscopy or open laparotomy for cholecystectomy. *Anesthesiology*, **77**: 4, 675-80.

Roberts C.J., Goodman N.W. (1990) Gastro-oesophageal reflux during elective laparoscopy. *Anaesthesia*, **45**, 1009–11.

Rose D.K.R., Cohen M.M., Soutter D.I. (1992) Laparoscopic cholecystectomy: the anaesthetist's point of view. *Canadian Journal of Anaesthesia*, **39**, 809–15.

Seed R.F., Shakespeare T.F., Muldoon M.J. (1970) Carbon dioxide homeostasis during anaesthesia for laparoscopy. *Anaesthesia*, **25**, 223–31.

Smith I., Ding Y., White P.F. (1992) Post-laparoscopic myalgias: effect of propofol, succinycholine and atracurium. *Anesthesiology*, **77**, A951.

Taylor E., Feinstein R., White P.F., Soper N. (1992) Anaesthesia for laparoscopic cholecystectomy. Is nitrous oxide contraindicated? *Anesthesiology*, **76**, 541–3.

Uhlich G.A. (1982) Laparoscopy: the question of the proper gas. *Gastrointestinal Endoscopy*, **28**, 212–13.

Watcha M.F., White P.F. (1992) Post-operative nausea and vomiting. *Anesthesiology*, **77**, 162–84.

Yacoub O.F., Cardona I., Coveler L.A., Dodson M.G. (1982) Carbon dioxide embolism during laparoscopy. *Anesthesiology*, **57**, 533-535.

6: Complications of Laparoscopy

M.J.COPTCOAT AND A.D.JOYCE

Introduction

Operative laparoscopy is minimally invasive and is associated with a low morbidity and rapid return to normal activities. But complications, although infrequent, can occur at any point of a laparoscopic procedure. The majority are minor and do not drastically alter the outcome, but on some rare occasions a minimally invasive concept is transformed into a maximally invasive emergency salvage procedure. Prevention is better than cure, and fortunately most complications can be nipped in the bud by the alert laparoscopist.

The complications of a laparoscopic cholecystectomy have been much discussed recently, and the stark fact is that common bile duct injury (and, in particular, stricture formation) during a laparoscopic cholecystectomy is many times more common than was seen following an open cholecystectomy. The conclusion is not that the procedure is inherently dangerous but that surgeons have not been adequately trained (Peters *et al.* 1991).

Before a resumé of possible laparoscopic complications and their management, let us focus on prevention, which in retrospect comes from adequate training. Operative laparoscopy is a quantum leap from even modern endourology, and experience needs to be gained with simulators and, ideally, *in vivo* rehearsal before patients are treated. Many laparoscopic procedures in urology follow the same basic protocol, especially techniques in the pelvis. There is, then, an overlap and consolidation of experience. But more advanced procedures such as a laparoscopic nephrectomy or pyeloplasty need specific training, and some form of preceptorship is preferred if early complications are to be kept to a minimum.

Two characteristics of laparoscopy in urology stand out at the present time. The first is that the surgeon's age is often inversely proportional to the surgeon's laparoscopic acumen and, second, our trainees have to learn from relatively inexperienced senior staff. Our gynaecological colleagues who have been immersed in laparoscopy, albeit mainly of the simple variety, do not have the same problems. Their advice to us is to overtrain through this chronological problem and we will witness future urologists just as adept at laparoscopy as at transurethral resection or open bladder reconstruction. Until this time, centres that specialize in laparoscopic work will continue to be the focus of work and training. But in one generation, the full breadth of laparoscopy in urology will be seen in every urology department.

It is too early in the development and learning of these new operative laparoscopic procedures to know the true incidence of complications. At the present time we can only look at a comparison with previous laparoscopic work in gynaecology (Table 6.1), with the cautionary note that most complications occur when the laparoscopic surgeon has performed fewer than 250 procedures. We are optimistic that this is not a figure to be highlighted in urology, because the instrumentation is safer, and we know from video TURP studies that the learning curve of an operator when he is constantly viewed is much more rapid.

The incidence of gynaecological laparoscopic-related morbidity is estimated to be less than 4% (Mintz 1977, Kane & Kreijs 1984). A summary of the morbidity in our first 150 cases at King's College Hospital appears in Table 6.2. Its urological total of 10% sits uncomfortably beside the previous gynaecological total of under 4%, but it includes a series of 43 laparoscopic nephrectomy cases. If this special group is excluded, the incidence of complications falls to 5.8%. Of our total complications for all laparoscopic procedures, only three cases were abandoned peroperatively. Two were for nonprogression of laparoscopic nephrectomies due to dense inflammatory adhesions associated with stone disease, and a third was a laparoscopic node dissection that had to be opened to control a bleeding point. Four cases of postoperative haemorrhage occurred after laparoscopic nephrectomies. These patients were explored with a laparotomy 4–12 hours postoperatively because of a fall in haemoglobin and a persistent tachycardia. Blood loss from a wound drain was not a reliable sign and it was disappointing to note that after completion of each of these laparoscopic nephrectomies, good haemostasis had been observed. Our feeling is that occult haemorrhage can occur below a thin puddle of clotted blood, and so meticulous irrigation, aspiration and, if necessary, swabbing of the renal bed are required before removing the ports.

Further specific complications will be covered in each procedure later in this book. General complications and their management will now be discussed.

Table 6.1 Incidence of complications of gynaecological laparoscopy (Phillips 1977)

Complication	Incidence %
Pneumoperitoneum-related	0.7
Haemorrhage	0.6
Perforating injuries	0.3
Infection	0.1
Intestinal burns	0.05
Cardiac arrest	0.03
Total	1.78

Table 6.2 Complications of laparoscopic urological surgery in 150 cases at King's College Hospital, London

Complication	Incidence	
Access		
Pneumoperitoneum		7
Perforating injuries	(4.6%)	
		0
Operative		
Haemorrhage		
Cardiac dysrhythmia		1
	(0.6%)	
Postoperative		
Local infections		1
Chest infections	(0.6%)	
Urinary retention		
Haemorrhage		0
		2
Total	(1.2%)	

Problems with access

Pneumoperitoneum

The choice of gases for establishing a pneumoperitoneum and the complications of carbon dioxide insufflation have been mentioned in Chapter 5.

The complications of Veress needle and trocar insertion have been greatly reduced by the use of disposable ports and needles with safety shields. An unusual complication of insufflation needle placement is massive distention of the preperitoneal space when the tip of the needle has not gone through into the peritoneum. This should be suspected if the injection of 5 ml of saline meets with resistance and initial insufflation pressures stay at the upper predetermined limit of 12 mmHg. Recognition of this problem sometimes only occurs with the introduction of the laparoscope. In these cases, the Veress needle should be inserted lateral to the rectus sheath, and similarly the first port should be placed well away from the now artificially thickened central abdominal wall. Initial intraperitoneal views will still seem cramped but this will disappear as the carbon dioxide is absorbed.

Abdomens that have undergone previous surgery or where one suspects intraperitoneal adhesions must be respected, and if there is any doubt that a free intra-abdominal space cannot be entered then an open minilaparotomy incision should be made and the first cannula with blunt trocar inserted as described by Hasson (1971). Subsequent port sitings can then be made under direct vision after preliminary adhesions have been divided. Routine placement of the first port in this way is recommended for those inexperienced in using a Veress needle, and it would certainly avoid the rare but catastrophic aortic perforation incident (Peterson *et al.* 1982).

Insufflation of carbon dioxide into the peritoneal cavity is sometimes associated with postoperative shoulder pain. This referred pain is believed to be the result of direct irritation of the diaphragm by carbon dioxide forming carbonic acid. It may occur in as many as one-third of patients, but is usually severe in fewer than 5%. Slow initial insufflation helps to reduce the complication but, if present, generally it will resolve spontaneously within 24 hours. Prolonged operative laparoscopic procedures are also associated with widespread surgical emphysema if the seals around the ports are not secure. Although dramatic, this is usually completely asymptomatic, but nurses and junior medical staff should be aware of its unimportant presence. It is exaggerated during and after laparoscopic pelvic lymphadenectomy with the formation of a pneumocele of the scrotum.

Trocar placement

A potential complication of trocar placement is a vascular injury within the abdominal wall. This may result in bleeding around the cannula and into the peritoneal cavity or the formation of an abdominal wall haematoma. The abdominal wall should be transilluminated with the laparoscope before incising the skin and inserting the trocar. If an arterial or venous injury does occur then the cannula should be left in place to tamponade the vessel and allow it to seal. All trocar insertion sites should be carefully examined prior to and after removal of the cannula.

If active bleeding is identified (this is usually from the superficial epigastric artery), a haemostatic suture can be placed with a hand needle through the abdominal wall or by passage of a Stamey needle under laparoscopic vision (Green *et al.* 1992).

The risk of a trocar injury to the gastrointestinal tract is very small in the absence of dense adhesions. However, bowel preparations are recommended during difficult cases when the bowel must be retracted in order for the surgeon to operate accurately. Gastrointestinal (Soderstrom & Levy 1986), vascular (Lynn *et al.* 1982) or urinary tract injuries (Deshmukh 1982) resulting from laparoscopic trocar insertion are rare (0.3%) and should be managed in the same way as any other penetrating injury to the abdomen.

Injury from an insufflation needle to a major blood vessel is unlikely to require an immediate laparotomy, providing that pressure can be applied from an associate blunt instrument. However, unlike insufflation-needle injuries, perforation of a major blood vessel with a trocar should be managed by immediate laparotomy and repair.

If the abdomen does need to be opened in an emergency, a safe but rapid technique is to pull the laparoscope up against the abdominal wall and cut down into it with a skin knife.

Endocoordination

Endocoordination is an important aspect of the laparoscopic surgical learning curve. The two-dimensional image produced by current laparoscopic video systems results in a loss of depth perception. This handicap can be partially overcome by adapting specific visual clues to assist in the proper placement and orientation of laparoscopic instruments. It is important to maintain continual visualization of the operating instruments on the video monitor. When the telescope is removed, all instruments should be kept stationary. It is this relative lack of depth perception that requires a long learning curve.

For the assistant, whose orientation is at 180° to the telescope and camera, the visual problem may be compounded by a monitor with a seemingly inverted image. The critical angle of a manipulation instrument to the field of vision is 90°. Anything less than 90°, and especially close to being parallel, proves to be easy, but an angle over 90° is a very difficult hand–brain challenge. If the problem is not artificially corrected on the monitor, assistants must consciously think about what they are doing rather than what it appears they may have to do with their instruments. Some find it easier to view the surgeon's monitor regardless of the position difficulties.

The bowel may be injured by diathermy, either directly or, very rarely, as a complication of capacitance discharge via a metal cannula that is insulated from the abdominal wall by a nonconductive grip. It is sometimes difficult to locate the exact point, and if injury is suspected, careful and gradual inspection from a standard reference point such as the caecum should be carried out, and any bowel injury should be oversewn. This can easily be accomplished with modern needle-holders and sutures.

Haemorrhage

The greatest problem facing laparoscopic surgeons is haemorrhage. It is rarely so severe as to require an emergency laparotomy, but on many occasions what might have been a trivial leak corrected by tamponade can produce an inoperative field. First, the bleeding tends to obscure the line of dissection. Second, blood absorbs light intensity with consequent reduction in vision. Attempted aspiration of blood can inadvertently remove the carbon dioxide from the operative space, and so it collapses. This in turn allows more blood to ooze, and what should have been a minor complication can lead to an unnecessary open laparotomy. Prevention is by anticipating any bleeding with the use of grasping forceps close to the site of dissection.

Any potential haemorrhage can be grasped by either the operator or the assistant. Then there is plenty of time to exchange instruments for either a clip applier or diathermy. The important practical point about applying clips is that one should always be able to see the ends approximate on the other side of the vessel. If a position cannot be identified then one must suspect that haemostasis will not be intact. Siting of the clip ends is also important to determine that they have not crept onto another associated structure. Many of the common bile duct injuries during a laparoscopic cholecystectomy have been due to misplacement of haemostatic clips.

References

Deshmukh A.S. (1982) Laparoscopic bladder injury. *Urology*, **19**, 306–7.

Green L.S., Loughlin K.R., Kavoussi L.R. (1992) Management of epigastric vessel injury during laparoscopy. *Journal of Endourology*, **6**: 2, 99-101.

Hasson H.M. (1971) A modified instrument and method for laparoscopy. *American Journal of Obstetrics and Gynaecolgy*, **110**: 6, 886–7.

Kane M.G., Kreijs G.J. (1984) Complications of diagnostic laparoscopy in Dallas: A seven-year prospective study. *Gastrointestinal Endoscopy*, **30**, 237–40.

Lynn S.C., Katz A.R., Ross P.J. (1982) Aortic perforation sustained at laparoscopy. *Journal of Reproductive Medicine*, **27**, 217–19.

Mintz M. (1977) Risks and prophylaxis in laparoscopy: A survey of 100,000 cases. *Journal of Reproductive Medicine*, **18**, 269–72.

Peters J.H., Ellison E.C., Innes J.T. *et al.* (1991) Safety and efficacy of laparoscopic cholecystectomy. *Annals of Surgery*, **213**, 3-12.

Peterson H.B., Greenspan J.R., Ory H.W. (1982) Death following puncture of the aorta during laparoscopic sterilization. *Obstetrics and Gynaecology*, **59**, 133–4.

Phillips J.M. (1977) Complications in laparoscopy. *International Journal of Gynaecology and Obstetrics*, **15**, 157–62.

Soderstrom R.M., Levy B.S. (1986) Bowel injuries during laparoscopy: Causes and medicolegal questions. *Continuing Obstetrics and Gynaecology*, **27**, 41-45.

7: The Metabolic Response to Operative Laparoscopy

C.G. EDEN AND M.J. COPTCOAT

Introduction

The explosion of interest in operative laparoscopy by surgeons and the public alike has resulted in an almost unique event in surgical history. With the notable exception of extracorporeal shockwave lithotripsy, no other treatment modality has been so widely and rapidly embraced without having first proven its safety and superiority in comparative clinical trials. There seems to be an intuitive feeling amongst the surgical fraternity, hitherto based largely on anecdotal evidence, that an operation performed through a small hole must somehow be better for the patient.

Balanced against the potential benefit of this minimal-access approach is the longer anaesthetic time for many laparoscopic operations, especially for complex procedures such as nephrectomy and ureterolysis. This is of concern, because we already know from sham operations on animals that a general anaesthetic alone elicits a stress response and from human studies that anaesthesia causes immune compromise (Platt *et al.* 1989).

The economic benefits of a laparoscopic approach in the context of gallbladder surgery are well established (Cuschieri *et al.* 1990): it allows an earlier discharge from hospital and return to work, in addition to a smaller postoperative analgesic requirement. However, little attention has been paid to determining how operative laparoscopy compares with open surgery at the biological level.

The metabolic response to trauma

Evolutionary selection pressures undoubtedly conferred some advantage on those seriously injured ancestors of ours whose metabolism could mobilize energy stores and retain water to aid healing whilst they were unable to forage.

An identical metabolic response is seen after modern surgery, but we now recognize that the hyperglycaemia, negative nitrogen balance, fluid retention and muscle weakness that result can be harmful, particularly in patients with little cardiorespiratory or nutritional reserve. The accompanying relative immunosupression leads to an increased susceptibility to exogenous and nosocomial infection (Chandra 1983), impaired wound-healing and tissue repair (Windsor *et al.* 1988) and, more worryingly, may adversely affect the results of surgery for malignancy.

Table 7.1 Mediators of the stress response (Wilmore 1991)

Hormone	Cytokine	Lipid
Glucagon	Tumour necrosis factor	Platelet-activating factor
Glucocorticoids	Interleukin-1 Interleukin-2 Thromboxane A2 Interleukin-6	
Catecholamines	Interferon gamma	Leucotriene B4
Arginine vasopressin	Prostaglandin E2	
Aldosterone		

Mediators of the stress response

The mediators of the stress response can be divided into three groups: hormones, cytokines and lipid mediators (Table 7.1). The pattern of mediator release depends on the stressful stimulus applied, and it appears that the three response systems are interconnected by amplification loops and negative-feedback systems (Wilmore 1991).

The role of carbon dioxide

The ready availability, low cost and inertness of carbon dioxide (CO_2) has made it the gas of choice for the creation and maintenance of a pneumoperitoneum. Its disadvantage lies in its great solubility in peritoneal fluid, forming carbonic acid. Intraoperative and early postoperative pooling of carbonic acid under the diaphragm and consequent diaphragmatic irritation is thought to be responsible for the postlaparoscopy pain syndrome, which is characterized by shoulder-tip pain.

The pain is more commonly felt on the right, probably due to trapping of fluid between the liver and the right hemidiaphragm. The chief practical problem caused by the great solubility of CO_2, however, is the generation of a metabolic acidosis caused by absorption of carbonic acid, even when the intraperitoneal pressure is continuously maintained below 12 mmHg.

This can lead to cardiac dysrhythmias and depression of cardiac output, and occasionally it necessitates conversion to an open procedure. Continuous monitoring of end-tidal CO_2 ($EtCO_2$) is therefore essential as it may be necessary to increase the minute-volume ventilation to maintain the $EtCO_2$ in the ideal range of 4.5–5.5%. This is particularly so during relatively long laparoscopic procedures such as nephrectomy.

The evidence presented by clinical studies

The hypothesis that it is less metabolically stressful to perform an operation with minimal trauma of access is an attractive one and is the basis for three recent studies which have sought to compare the metabolic responses to a laparoscopic operation with its open counterpart. Two of the studies have compared laparoscopic with open cholecystectomy and the third (Eden & Coptcoat, submitted for publication) has investigated nephrectomy. In addition, a fourth study (Frazee *et al.* 1991) has compared postoperative lung function in patients undergoing laparoscopic and open cholecystectomy.

Laparoscopic cholecystectomy

McMahon *et al.* (1993) compared laparoscopic cholecystectomy with open cholecystectomy performed through a conventional upper midline incision, whilst Mealy *et al.* (1992) used a 5–7 cm minilaparotomy incision. All patients underwent elective surgery. McMahon's group analysed venous blood taken at regular intervals during the first postoperative week for C-reactive protein, interleukin-6, cortisol, albumin, transferrin, iron, fibrinogen, fibrin degradation products, polymorphonuclear elastase, white cell, neutrophil and lymphocyte count. Twenty-four-hour urine collections were analysed for urea, creatinine, 3-methylhistidine and catecholamines. They found that although there was a wide interpersonal variation in the magnitude of the stress response there was no statistically significant difference between the two groups of 10 patients in any of the parameters measured. Mealy investigated the metabolic response to surgery in 21 patients (10 undergoing laparoscopic and 11 open surgery), in addition to assessing postoperative lung function and pain perception using a linear analogue scale. The metabolic parameters measured were urinary cortisol, vanillylmandelic acid (VMA), metanephrines and nitrogen loss, serum complement component C_3 and C-reactive protein (CRP), full blood count and erythrocyte sedimentation rate (ESR). Lung function was assessed by spirometry, peak-flowmetry and arterial blood gas sampling. Statistically significant differences were seen between the two groups in respect of urinary VMA excretion (higher in the laparoscopic group), ESR and CRP values (higher in the open group). Postoperative lung function tests demonstrated a significantly lower pH and higher $P\text{CO}_2$ in the open group, indicating poorer respiratory performance. The postoperative analgesic requirement was also significantly greater in the open group. In a study of 36 consecutive patients undergoing elective cholecystectomy using either a right subcostal incision (16 patients) or a four-port technique (20 patients), Frazee *et al.* (1991) measured lung function using body plethysmography and a flow-volume loop. The distribution of smokers was roughly equal between the two groups. Lung function tests performed both prior to and 24 hours after surgery showed that all three parameters measured—forced vital capacity (*FVC*), forced expiratory volume at 1 second (FEV_1) and forced expiratory flow 25–75%)—were significantly higher following surgery in the laparoscopic group.

Laparoscopic nephrectomy

In the authors' still unpublished study, 14 consecutive patients undergoing nephrectomy were studied: seven patients in the open group and seven in the laparoscopic group. Patients in the open group underwent nephrectomy via a loin (six patients) or a subcostal approach (one patient): three patients for benign disease and four for malignancy. In the laparoscopic group a five-port transperitoneal ureter-first technique was used for nephrectomy in all seven patients. This involved a preliminary full-length ipsilateral colonic mobilization. Five patients had benign disease and two had a renal malignancy. Arterial blood was regularly sampled in the first 48 hours following surgery for estimation of white count, glucose and blood gases. Twenty-four-hour urine collections were used to measure urea, cortisol and catecholamine excretion at 0, 24, 48 and 168 hours following surgery. Lung function was assessed by spirometry and peakflowmetry prior to surgery and at 24 and 48 hours following surgery.

As in the patients undergoing cholecystectomy, there was no statistical difference in serum glucose, white cell count or urinary urea excretion between the laparoscopic and open groups. However, in contrast to the cholecystectomy patients, there was a significantly higher and more prolonged cortisol rise in the open cases (Fig. 7.1) and although the urinary adrenalin excretion (Fig. 7.2) was higher in the laparoscopic group at 24 hours, it fell more rapidly and was lower

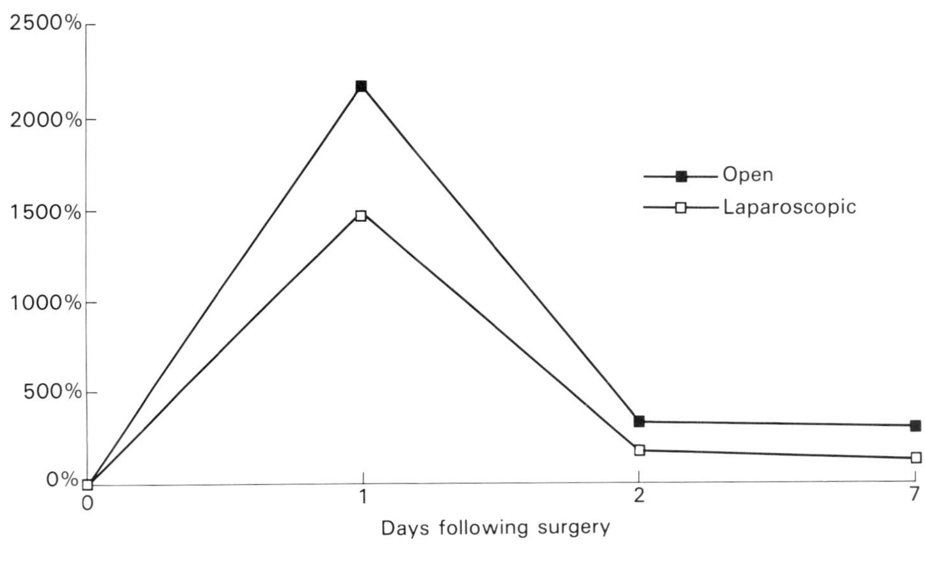

Fig. 7.1 Percentage change in 24-hour urinary cortisol excretion following nephrectomy. There was a significantly higher and more prolonged cortisol rise during an open nephrectomy than a laparoscopic nephrectomy.

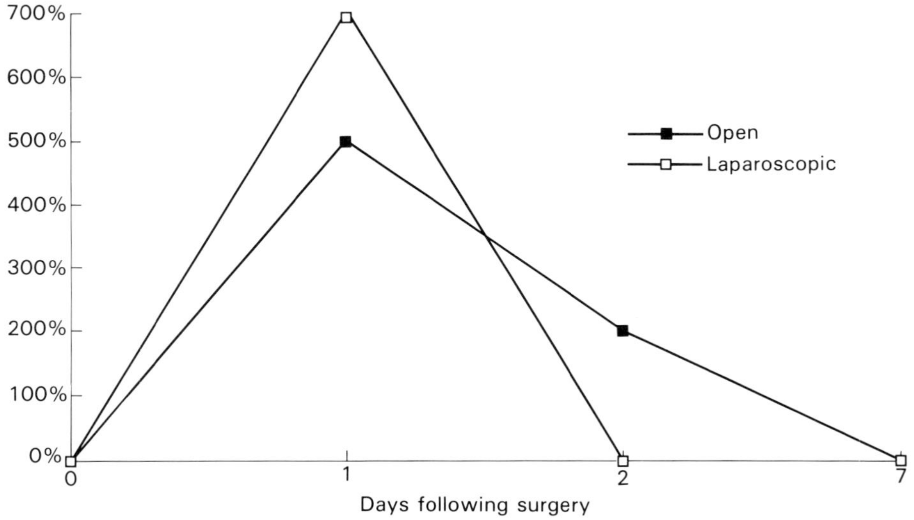

Fig. 7.2 Percentage change in 24-hour urinary adrenalin excretion. The excretion was higher after a laparoscopic nephrectomy until 24 hours postoperatively. Then it fell more rapidly and was lower than in the open group by 48 hours following surgery.

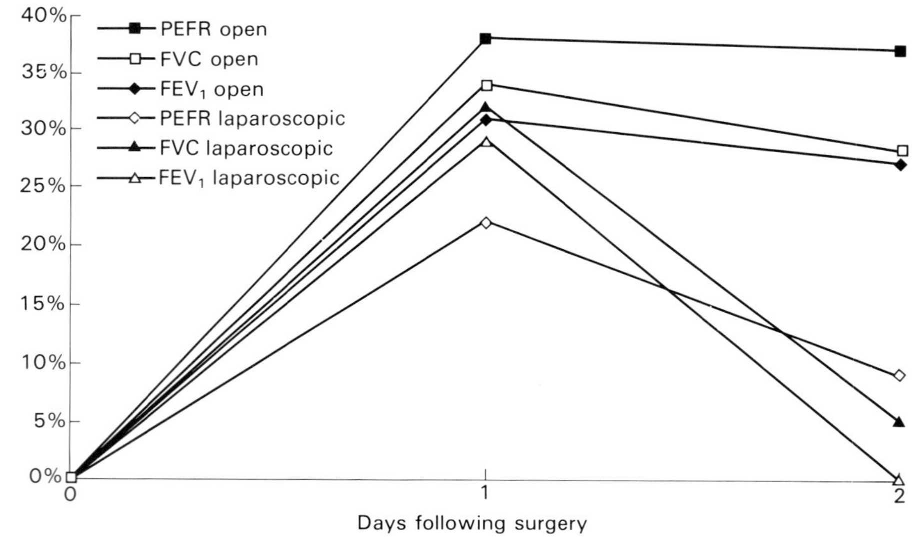

Fig. 7.3 Percentage reduction in lung function following nephrectomy. Postoperative pulmonary function as assessed by spirometry and peak-flowmetry were better preserved in the laparoscopic nephrectomy group.

than in the open group by 48 hours following surgery. Postoperative pulmonary function, as assessed by spirometry and peak-flowmetry, were better preserved in the laparoscopic group (Fig. 7.3). There was no significant difference between the two groups in respect of arterial blood gases, urinary noradrenalin or dopamine excretion.

The metabolic response to operative laparoscopy

It is interesting to speculate why there appears to be little metabolic advantage in performing a laparoscopic rather than an open cholecystectomy, whereas performing nephrectomy via a laparoscopic approach seems to elicit a significantly smaller stress response than by open operation. Access to the gallbladder by any of the standard open approaches requires much less tissue trauma than does open nephrectomy, which usually involves the division of a considerable bulk of muscle. It is perhaps not too surprising, therefore, that the metabolic consequences of performing the same operation using a minimal access approach are similar in the case of cholecystectomy but dissimilar in the case of nephrectomy. It appears that a laparoscopic approach to an operation in which the creation of access for its open counterpart involves substantial tissue trauma (such as nephrectomy) may be biologically superior. Conversely, the results also suggest that a minimal-access alternative to open procedures, such as minilap cholecystectomy and herniorrhaphy, in which the trauma of access is not dissimilar to that in the insertion of three or four trocars, cannot be justified on the grounds that it provokes a smaller stress response, unless it results in superior postoperative pulmonary function. The former operation fulfils these criteria, but the latter clearly does not.

Catecholamines

Two major pathways seem to be responsible for initiating and maintaining the stress response (Wilmore 1991): neural stimuli (which can be abolished by epidural anaesthesia (Brandt *et al.* 1978) and humoral factors (Table 7.1). It is interesting to note that the urinary VMA and adrenalin excretion was higher in the first 24 hours following laparoscopic cholecystectomy and nephrectomy, respectively, than in the open group. The cause may be increased afferent nerve impulse traffic to the pituitary–adrenal axis caused by stimulation of peritoneal stretch receptors by the pneumoperitoneum. The hypothesis is supported by the observation that the mean adrenalin excretion in the laparoscopic nephrectomy group during the second 24-hour period fell back to within the normal range (Fig. 7.2). A study of a further cohort of patients undergoing laparoscopic cholecystectomy, with half of the patients randomized to receive epidural anaesthesia and the other half not, is therefore indicated to further investigate this theory. In the case of the laparoscopic nephrectomy patients, an additional mechanism may be responsible for the findings: intraoperative adrenalin release by the adrenals during mobilization of the superior pole of the kidney, which is a difficult laparoscopic manoeuvre.

Cortisol

Horgan *et al.* (1992) have shown that laparoscopy is less immunotraumatic than open surgery by assessing spontaneous lymphocyte proliferation and responses to the mitogen phytohaemagglutinin in the cultured spleens of mice which had undergone laparotomy or laparoscopy. They also found higher mortality following infection with lipopolysaccharide in the laparoscopic group. These differences in immunity may be explained in part by the lower endogenous cortisol

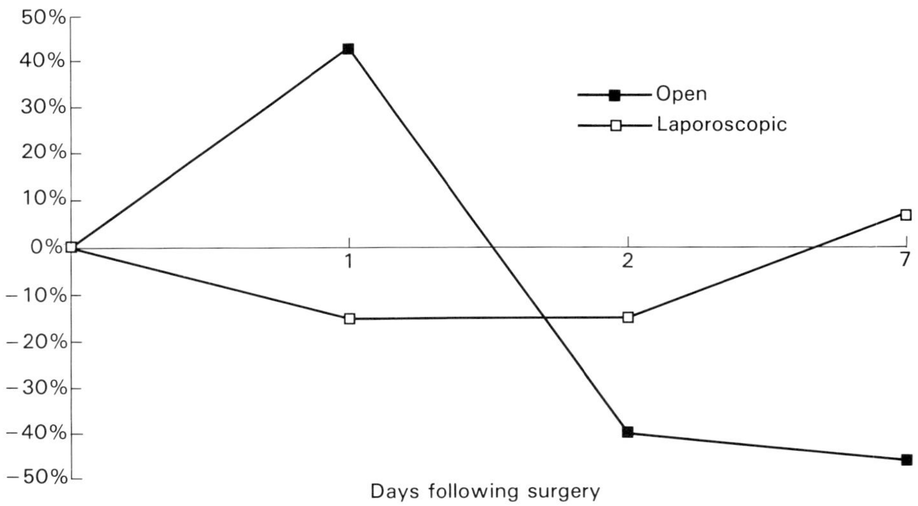

Fig. 7.4 Percentage change in 24-hour urinary urea excretion following both a laparoscopic and open nephrectomy. The differences are difficult to interpret, but it is likely that an improved post-operative hydration and reduced catabolism due to malignancy in the open nephrectomy group were responsible for the decline in the urea excretion seen in both groups.

secretion in the laparoscopic group, as noted in the authors' study. This has potential implications with regard to postoperative fluid retention, infection, wound-healing and, perhaps most importantly, recurrence following surgery for malignancy.

Nitrogen balance

The changes in perioperative urea excretion (Fig. 7.4) in the two nephrectomy groups are difficult to interpret. It seems likely that improved postoperative hydration and reduced catabolism due to malignancy were responsible for the decline in the urea excretion seen in the two groups. Assessment of the degree of catabolism by measurement of urinary urea excretion therefore seems to be inaccurate and further comment is inappropriate.

Calculation of nitrogen balance in patients whose hydration state is monitored by measurement of haematocrit and central venous pressure would give a better objective assessment of nitrogen flux, but one could still not control for errors due to the subclinical sepsis and malignant catabolism in many of the patients studied.

Generally, those patients who undergo minimal-access abdominal surgery have a much shorter, or absent, paralytic ileus, and they resume an oral diet sooner, than their conventionally operated counterparts. This constitutes an important difference between the two groups in the light of Windsor *et al.* (1988), who showed that recent food intake is more important than nutritional status for sound wound-healing.

Pulmonary function and pain perception

An upper abdominal wound typically results in a reduction of *FVC* and FEV_1 by 50% or more. These changes are caused by alteration of chest and abdominal wall dynamics and a decrease in lung volume due to basal atalectasis, respectively.

Diaphragmatic dysfunction following upper abdominal surgery is caused by splinting, due mainly to paralytic ileus, and paradoxical movement with respiration can occur. The pooled data from the three relevant studies confirms what common sense dictates, namely that the avoidance of a painful upper abdominal wound results in a lower postoperative analgesic requirement and better-preserved lung function. It also enables earlier postoperative patient mobilization and so reduces the likelihood of deep venous thrombosis and pulmonary embolism.

This has clear implications for patients with limited cardiorespiratory reserves. There can be no better example of this than the 101 kg patient in the laparoscopic nephrectomy series who had a mean reduction of only 19% in the three lung function parameters at 24 hours and 0% at 48 hours following operation. She would certainly have required thoracic epidural anaesthesia to allow acceptable gas exchange in the initial postoperative period had she undergone open surgery. The superior postoperative lung function should translate into a lower incidence of respiratory complications. Indeed, the only patient in the nephrectomy series who had a clinically apparent pulmonary complication (a hypoxic confusional state due to basal atalectasis) had undergone open nephrectomy.

The future

It is possible that the smaller stress response to laparoscopic nephrectomy results not only from less traumatic access, but also from gentler handling of tissues, and perhaps there is a lesson for us to learn here, which we can apply to our open surgical practice. Pharmacological and immune manipulation of the metabolic response to surgery may enable us to combine the excellent postoperative pulmonary function that follows operative laparoscopy with significantly decreased catabolism, fluid retention, muscle weakness, hyperglycaemia, and immunosupression, thus providing the ideal conditions for convalescence.

Nonsteroidal anti-inflammatory drugs have been shown (Wilmore, 1991) to reduce the effects of the cytokine interleukin-2, and studies are currently under way to investigate this effect in critically ill patients. Administration of monoclonal antibodies to other mediators of the stress response, such as tumour necrosis factor (Tracey *et al.* 1987), and platelet-activating factor (Sun & Hsueh 1988) also show great promise, as do insulin-like growth factor I (Guler *et al.* 1988) and epidermal growth factor (Brown *et al.* 1989), which have powerful anabolic properties.

Whatever the future of operative laparoscopy, it promises to be an exciting time for all those concerned with it. The greatest challenge that confronts us now is to devise laparoscopic operations that are both technically and biologically better that those attainable by today's open surgery.

References

Brandt M.R., Fernandes A., Mordhorst R. and Kehlet H. (1978) Epidural analgesia improves post-operative nitrogen balance. *British Medical Journal*, **1**, 1106–8.

Brown G.L., Nanney L.B., Griffen J. *et al.* (1989) Enhancement of wound healing by topical treatment with epidermal growth factor. *New England Journal of Medicine*, **321**, 76-9.

Chandra R.K. (1983) Nutrition, immunity and infection: present knowledge and future direction. *The Lancet*, **1**, 688–91.

Cuschieri A., Berci G., McSherry C.K. (1990) Laparoscopic cholecystectomy. *American Journal of Surgery*, **159**, 273.

Eden C.G. & Coptcoat M.J. (submitted for publication) The stress response to laparoscopic and open nephrectomy. *Journal of Minimally Invasive Therapy.*

Frazee R.C., Roberts J.W., Okeson G.C., *et al.* (1991) Open versus laparoscopic cholecystectomy. A comparison of postoperative pulmonary function. *Annals of Surgery*, **213**, 651–4.

Guler H.P., Zapf J., Froesch E.R. (1988) Recombinant human insulin-like growth factor I stimulates growth and has distinct effects on organ size in hypophysectomized rats. *Proceedings of the National Academy of Science of the USA*, **85**, 4889–93.

Horgan P.G., Fitzpatrick M., Couse N.F., Gorey T.F., Fitzpatrick J.M. (1992) Laparoscopy is less immunotraumatic than laparotomy. *Journal of Minimally Invasive Therapy*, **1**, 241–4.

Mealy K., Gallagher H., Barry M., Lennon F., Traynor O., Hyland J. (1992) Physiological and metabolic responses to open and laparoscopic cholecystectomy. *British Journal of Surgery*, **79**, 1061–4.

McMahon A.J., O'Dwyer P.J., Cruickshank A. *et al.* (1993) Metabolic changes after laparoscopic and minilap cholecystectomy: a randomised trial. Presentation at the annual meeting of the Surgical Research Society.

Platt M.P.W., Lovat P.E., Watson J.G., Aynsley-Green A. (1989) The effects of anaesthesia and surgery on lymphocyte populations and function in infants and children. *Journal of Pediatric Surgery*, **24**, 884–7.

Sun X.M. & Hsueh W. (1988) Bowel necrosis induced by tumour necrosis factor in rats is mediated by platelet-activating factor. *Journal of Clinical Investigations*, **81**, 1328–31.

Tracey K.J., Fong Y., Hesse D.G. *et al.* (1987) Anti-cachectin/TNF monoclonal antibodies prevent septic shock during lethal bacteraemia. *Nature*, **330**, 662–4.

Wilmore D.W. (1991) Catabolic illness. Strategies for enhancing recovery. *New England Journal of Medicine*, **325**, 695–702.

Windsor J.A., Knight G.S., Hill G.L. (1988) Wound healing response in surgical patients: recent food intake is more important than nutritional status. *British Journal of Surgery*, **75**, 135–7.

8: Laparoscopy for the Nonpalpable Testicle

M.J. COPTCOAT

Introduction

Laparoscopy acquired its first urological converts when it was realized that the nonpalpable testicle is best identified with laparoscopy, when often ultrasound or even computerized tomography is unhelpful (Weiss & Seashore 1987). Not only can the intra-abdominal testicle be found but, as is more common, the spermatic vessels can be followed down into the inguinal ring and this allows a subsequent accurate open exploration.

It was a logical step to utilize various operative laparoscopic techniques for biopsy or to remove such testicles (Thomas *et al.* 1992). A refinement in both instruments and techniques has allowed us to go one stage further and carry out a two-step orchidopexy with preliminary laparoscopic clip ligation of the spermatic vessels (Elder 1989, Bloom 1991).

Laparoscopic instrumentation

1 High-flow carbon dioxide insufflator
2 CCD camera and at least one monitor
3 Veress needle (safety)
4 0° 10mm laparoscope (300 optional)
5 Three 10mm ports with grips and converters/downsizers
6 Laparoscopic curved microscissors (diathermy connection)
7 Laparoscopic soft grasping forceps
8 Laparoscopic curved dissecting forceps
9 Endoclip* Applier (small/medium)

Technique

1 Under a general anaesthetic with muscle paralysis and assisted ventilation, the patient is put in a supine position with a 20–25° head-down tilt (Fig. 4.1a). A catheter is not usually required if the patient's bladder has recently emptied. Hip flexion is not required.
2 Formation of the pneumoperitoneum. The Veress needle is inserted at an angle of 45° into the empty pelvis (Fig. 4.2a). The position should be checked by aspiration and infusion of 5ml of saline, and during insufflation the intra-abdominal pressure should remain below

*A trademark of the United States Surgical Corporation (AutoSuture).

12 ml of mercury. In the hands of inexperienced laparoscopists, the disposable Veress needles with safety shield are safer. Previous major abdominal surgery is a relative contraindication. A previous appendicectomy is unlikely to have produced difficult intra-abdominal adhesions but anything more significant than this may produce an unnecessarily difficult procedure out of proportion to the open alternatives for the nonpalpable testicle.

3 Three 10 mm ports are placed according to the diagram (Fig. 8.1). The subumbilical port is for the telescope. The two secondary ports inserted along the lateral edges of the rectus sheath are for manipulative and dissecting instruments. The use of two 10 mm secondary ports allows the clip applicator to be introduced through either of these ports. The ports should be fixed with either grips or purse-string sutures.

4 The operator stands on the contralateral side of the patient whilst the camera-holder remains on the ipsilateral side.

5 The monitors should be at the bottom corners of the operating table (Fig. 8.2).

6 Adhesions to the sigmoid colon may need to be divided on the left-hand side before the testicular vessels become evident. The internal inguinal ring should be inspected first, because a small dysplastic testicle that has not been evident on CT or ultrasound may be sitting

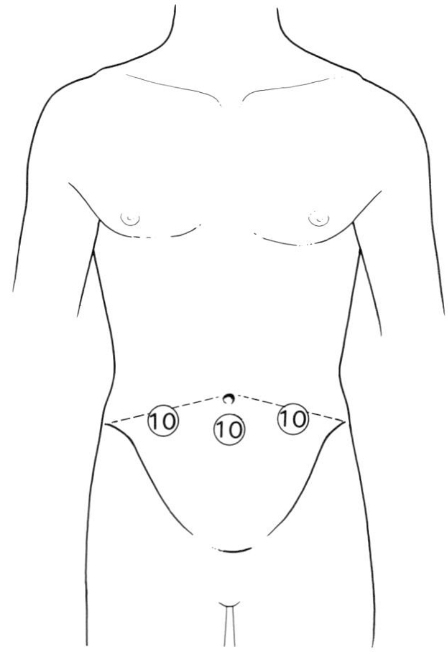

Fig. 8.1 The sites for the three 10 mm ports for a laparoscopic abdominal orchidectomy.

Fig. 8.2 The layout of equipment for a laparoscopic abdominal orchidectomy.

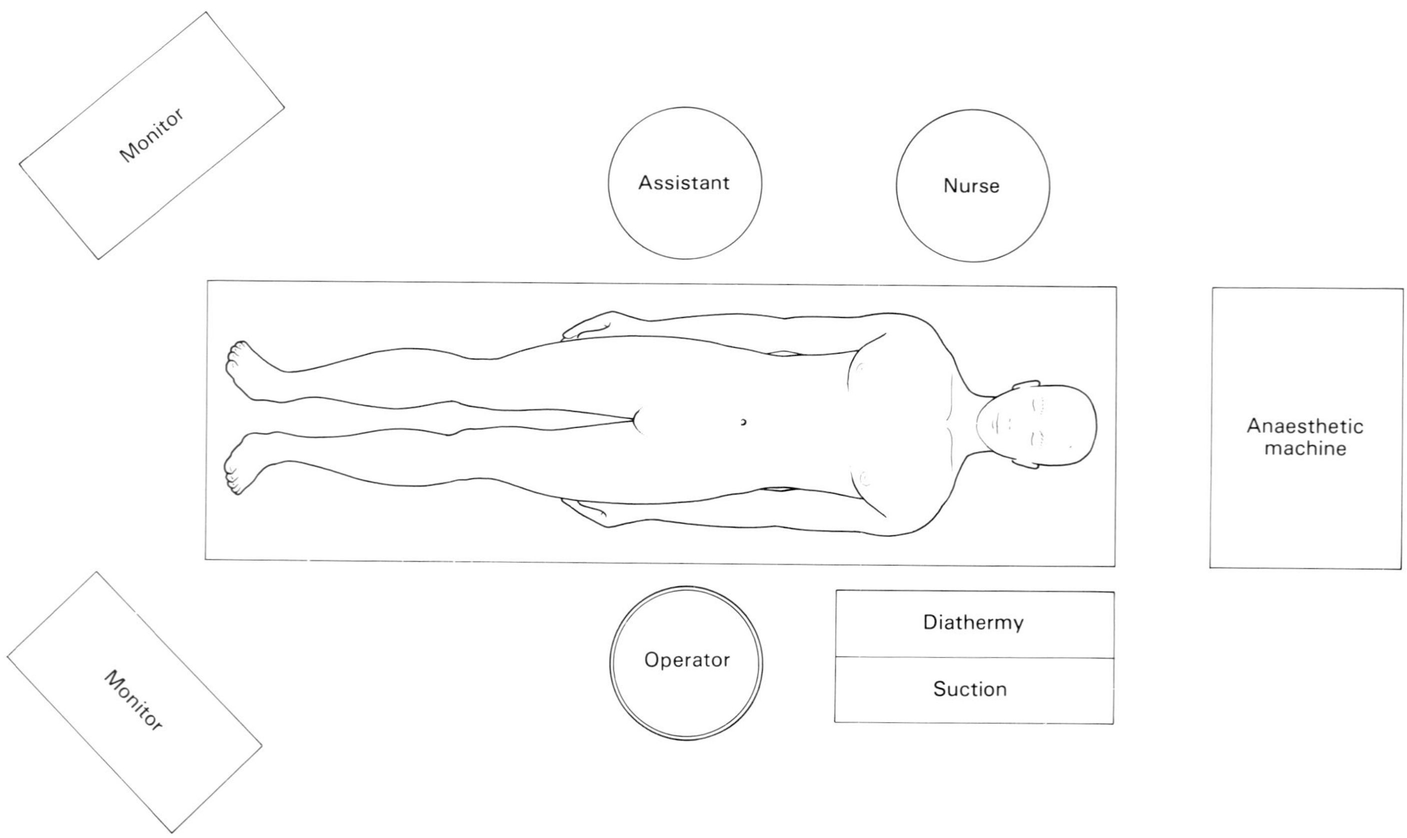

just inside the inguinal canal. The testicular vessels are a constant guide to the site of the testicle and it is only when they have been followed to their termination that one can conclude a complete absence when appropriate.

7 The patient's age and an assessment of the testicle's normality will determine the next step.

(a) If the testicle requires excision then the testicular vessels should be divided between pairs of clips (Fig. 8.3). The testicle can usually be drawn by forceps into the cannula of one of the ports and removed with the port at the end of the procedure. If the testicle is larger than 10 mm then the port incision will have to be enlarged and the testicle removed directly through this. Such operations require minimal dissection and haemostasis is only rarely a problem.

(b) The first stage of a Fowler–Stephens orchidopexy can be carried out laparoscopically. Once the intra-abdominal testicle has been identified and recognized as normal, a laparoscopic biopsy can be taken for frozen section if there is any doubt. The testicular artery and veins are divided between pairs of clips. Approximately six weeks after the first operation, the second but open stage of the orchidopexy can be carried out because the testicle will usually have retained an adequate blood supply from the artery to the vas.

8 The ports must be removed under direct vision. All carbon dioxide is evacuated.

9 To prevent wound-herniation, all wounds require a deep fascial suture. The skin can be sutured with a subcuticular absorbable suture or steristrips (Fig. 4.11); 3–5 ml of 0.5% marcaine are infiltrated into

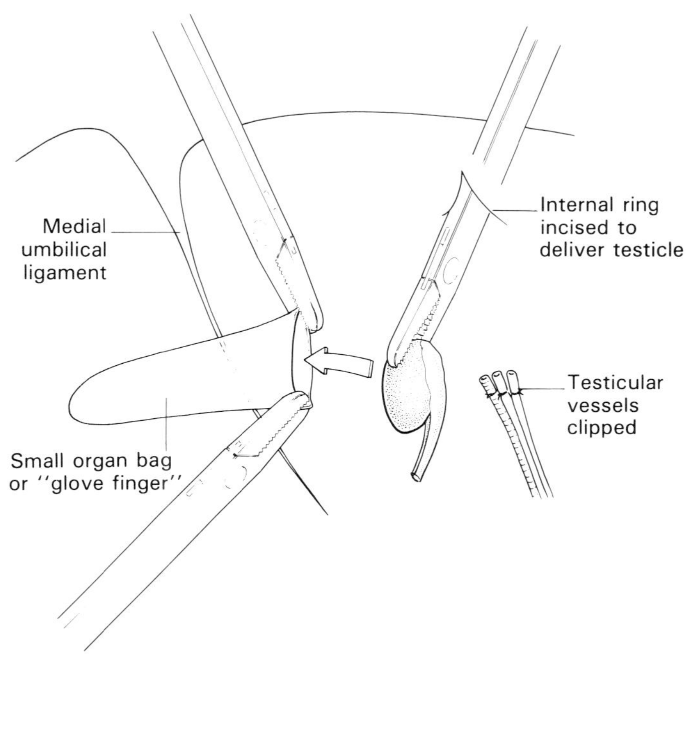

Fig 8.3 The testicular vessels to a dysplastic testicle just inside the internal inguinal ring have been clipped. The testicle is delivered into a small organ-retrieval bag or the finger from a large sterile surgical glove.

each wound. Patients require 1–2 hours hospitalization and can then be discharged home.

Discussion

Intra-abdominal cryptorchidism affects 8–9% of the cryptorchid population. It is generally accepted that these intra-abdominal testicles have a four-fold increased risk of malignancy compared to inguinal testicles and a 20–46-fold increased risk of malignancy compared to scrotal testicles. Additionally there is a significant increase in the number of germ-cell tumours encountered in unilateral cryptorchid testicles in patients who undergo orchidopexy after the age of 10. By the age of 10, the malignant potential of an intra-abdominal testicle outweighs the cosmetic benefit of orchidopexy. Prophylactic orchidectomy is appropriate therefore after this age and some have even suggested this protocol for children of more than six years of age. At whatever age orchidectomy is performed, the laparoscopic alternative is much less painful and results in a much more rapid return to normal activities.

Selective arteriography is an alternative diagnostic method for identifying an intra-abdominal testicle. It is less invasive than laparoscopy but carries the distinct disadvantage of being only a diagnostic tool: no further therapeutic action can be taken. Laparoscopy is slightly more invasive and requires a general anaesthetic but at least the testicle can either be excised or the spermatic vessels clipped to allow a second-stage orchidopexy.

References

Elder J.S. (1989) Laparoscopy and Fowler–Stephens orchidopexy in the management of the impalpable testis. *Urological Clinics of North America*, **16**: 2, 399–411.

Bloom D. (1991) Two-step orchiopexy with pelvioscopic clip ligation of spermatic vessels. *Journal of Urology*, **145**, 1030–3.

Thomas M.D., Mercer L.C., Saltzein E.C. (1992) Laparoscopic orchidectomy for unilateral intra-abdominal testis. *Journal of Urology*, **148**, 1251–3.

Weiss R.M. & Seashore J.H. (1987) Laparoscopy in the management of the nonpalpable testis. *Journal of Urology*, **138**, 344–82.

9: Laparoscopic Varicocelectomy

M.J. COPTCOAT AND A.D. JOYCE

Introduction

A varicocele is an abnormal tortuosity and dilatation of the testicular veins within the spermatic cord. A varicocele is found in approximately 15% of the general population and in at least 35% of infertile men (Greenberg 1977). It is also clear, however, that not all varicoceles are associated with abnormalities of the semen. Varicoceles do not occur with equal frequency on the left and right sides, as approximately 90% are left-sided.

Differences in the venous drainage patterns on the right and left testicular veins may account for this left-sided predominance. The left testicular vein drains into the left renal vein whereas the right testicular vein drains into the inferior vena cava.

In addition, there is a higher incidence of absent venous valves in the left side than in the right (Ahlberg *et al.* 1966). Unilateral right-sided varicoceles are uncommon. They raise the possibility of thrombosis or occlusion of the vena cava or situs inversus. Approximately 10% of patients present to infertility clinics with bilateral varicoceles, but the incidence may be much higher if epidemiological studies were repeated with doppler ultrasound rather than depending on the clinical findings alone.

Patients with a varicocele can present with testicular growth retardation in adolescence or as an adult with either subfertility or symptoms of a dragging discomfort in the scrotum. The latter presentation can be successfully managed by various methods of ligation or occlusion of the dilated testicular veins. It is unusual for any such procedure not to remove the symptoms even though there is a varied but high incidence of residual and recurrent varicocele.

One presumes that the venous congestion has at least been lowered below a threshold at which symptoms of discomfort are experienced. However, such a therapeutic strategy is not suitable for the patient with a varicocele who presents with subfertility. This group of patients deserve the procedure that completely abolishes the varicocele, has the least recurrence rate and is associated with improved male fertility.

Traditional approaches to the surgical repair of a varicocele include retroperitoneal (Palomo 1949) and inguinal (Ivanissevich 1960) operations. A hydrocele is a major complication of these operations. Szabo & Kessler (1984) reviewed the incidence of hydrocele formation after varicocelectomy and found rates varying from 3% to 39%, and in their own series an incidence of 7.2%. The protein concentration of the hydrocele fluid indicated that lymphatic obstruction was the cause of hydrocele formation after varicocelectomy.

Testicular atrophy is the most devastating complication of varicocelectomy, but it is rarely reported and its true incidence is unknown. Human studies suggest that ligation of the testicular artery is associated with a substantial risk of testicular injury during orchidopexy but this may only be relevant to those varicocele ligations within the inguinal canal. The high Palomo approach probably avoids this complication because testicular artery interruption takes place above the vas and its own arterial supply, which will act as a potential collateral source to the testicle. However, even a relative decrease in arterial flow may affect spermatogenesis without overt atrophy or morphological changes.

The incidence of persistent or recurrent varicocele following surgical repair in adults varies from 5% to 45% (Rothman *et al.* 1981, Belgrano *et al.* 1984) and appears to be even more common after repair of the paediatric varicocele. Venography of recurrent varicoceles has revealed that most recurrences are the result of midretroperitoneal or low inguinal parallel collaterals (Sayfan *et al.* 1981, Murray *et al.* 1986) but 7% of all recurrences appear to be due to scrotal collaterals (Kaufman *et al.* 1983).

Attempts at decreasing the complication rates following varicocelectomy have led to the development of microsurgical approaches which have the advantages of identification and preservation of the testicular artery and lymphatics and decrease the incidence of hydrocele formation and testicular artery injury. Intraoperative venography performed at the time of conventional varicocelectomy identifies the venous collaterals but markedly increases the operating time and still results in a significant incidence of varicocele recurrence similar to the disappointing results of percutaneous embolization (Kaufman *et al.* 1983, Porst *et al.* 1984).

Goldstein *et al.* (1992) have recently brought these issues into focus and has described a technique of open microsurgical (x 8 magnification) varicocelectomy with delivery of the testicle, division of gubernacular vessels, sparing of the testicular artery and lymphatics: 640 of these procedures were carried out in 429 men. Among 382 men available for follow-up examination from six months to seven years postoperatively, no hydroceles and no cases of testicular atrophy were found.

A total of four unilateral recurrent varicoceles (0.6%) was identified. Four scrotal haematomas occurred (0.6%) but no other complications. Preoperative and postoperative semen analyses were obtained in 271 men. They showed a statistically significant increase in sperm count, in motility and in normal forms. The pregnancy rate was 43% of couples followed for a minimum of six months postoperatively.

These results are vastly superior to previously reported alternative procedures and if reproducible by others should become the gold standard for varicocelectomy techniques.

The laparoscopic varicocelectomy is one of the most commonly performed laparoscopic procedures in urology departments but its clinical role has been much less clear than its use in exposing urologists to relatively straightforward operative laparoscopy. However, it has suffered from the early concept of trying to copy by laparoscopic means an established open procedure; in this case, the high Palomo testicular vein ligation. The most effective laparoscopic varicocelectomy technique must produce results similar to those reported by Goldstein and still have clear-cut advantages in minimizing the trauma of access and the delay in returning to normal activities.

The current laparoscopic telescopes and imaging systems have a potential magnification factor of up to three times. This has often been a disadvantage to the surgeon who is not used to having his or her nose right up against the object. But it should now be exploited as a form of internal operating microscope. In this respect it can be used to identify closely the testicular vessels beneath the peritoneum. Lymphatic and testicular artery ligation can be avoided whilst the spermatic vessels are left *in situ* free of tension because there is no need to bring them up to the surface. Such accurate dissection demands attention to the precise anatomy of the spermatic vessels (a recurrent theme in laparoscopy), where anatomical layers or linings are better appreciated and can be dissected more precisely than at open surgery.

Anatomy of the spermatic vessels

Beck *et al.* (1992), using an operating microscope with x 8 magnification have shown that the testicular veins and artery run within the internal spermatic fascia.

In 79 of 115 ligations (69%), a solitary testicular artery was identified. Two arteries were found in 27% and three arteries in 4% of men. In 50% of the 79 spermatic cords with a single testicular artery, the artery was adherent to the posterior surface of a large internal spermatic vein.

In 16 of the 31 cases in which two testicular arteries were identified, the artery was within two separate complexes of veins. Beck also describes an average of 3.6 (range 1–8) lymphatics within the internal spermatic fascia, a dilated vasal vein in 7% of cases and a dilated external spermatic vein separate from the spermatic cord and perforating the floor of the inguinal canal in 37% of cases.

Thus the laparoscopic varicocelectomy must be carried out in a meticulous way, avoiding the testicular arterial supply and, where possible, the lymphatics. The vas should be inspected for a dilated vasal vein and the peritoneum should be opened behind the inguinal canal to exclude a dilated external spermatic vein. The enclosing fascial sheaths require sharp, precise dissection which is best performed with fine scissors.

One cannot identify the gubernacular vessels during a laparoscopic varicocelectomy but their role is still unclear and should be left to provide venous drainage from the testicle through veins unaffected by the pathophysiological defect of a varicocele.

Instrumentation

1 High-flow carbon dioxide insufflator
2 CCD camera and at least one monitor
3 Veress needle (safety)
4 0° 10mm laparoscope (30° optional)
5 Three 10mm ports with grips and converters/downsizers
6 Laparoscopic curved microscissors (diathermy connection)
7 Laparoscopic soft grasping forceps
8 Laparoscopic curved dissecting forceps
9 Endoclip* Applier (small)

Technique

1 Under a general anaesthetic with muscle paralysis and assisted ventilation, the patient is put in a supine position with a 20–25° head-down tilt (Fig. 4.1a). A catheter is not usually required if the patient's bladder has recently emptied. Hip flexion is not required.
2 Formation of the pneumoperitoneum (Fig. 4.1): the Veress needle is inserted at an angle of 45° into the empty pelvis. The position should be checked by aspiration and infusion of 5ml of saline. The intra-abdominal pressure should remain below 12ml of mercury during insufflation. In the hands of inexperienced laparoscopists, the disposable Veress needles with a safety shield are safer. Previous major abdominal surgery is a relative contraindication. A previous appendicectomy is unlikely to have produced difficult intra-abdominal adhesions, but anything more significant than this may produce an unnecessarily difficult procedure out of proportion to the open alternatives that remain for a varicocelectomy. The Veress needle should be inserted through a subumbilical incision in an unscarred abdomen but in the presence of an appendicectomy scar, it is wise either to insert the Veress needle at the lateral edge of the left rectus sheath where one of the secondary ports would normally be placed, or to introduce the first port with a Hasson cut-down technique in this lateral position.

*A trademark of the United States Surgical Corporation (AutoSuture).

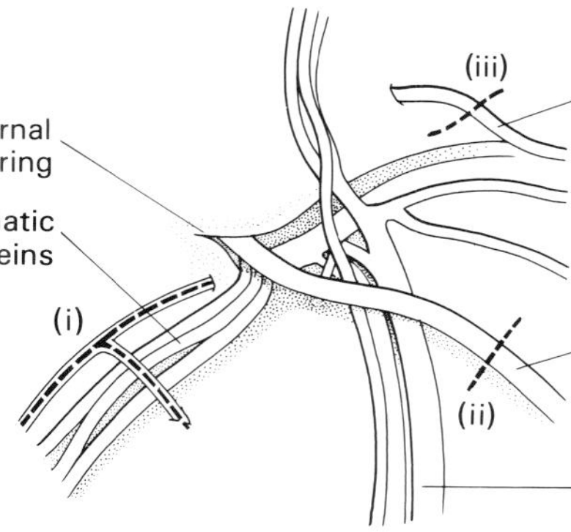

Fig. 9.1 The anatomy of the pelvic venous drainage from a varicocele, including (i) the internal spermatic veins, (ii) the vasal vein (iii) the external spermatic vein, and the peritoneal incisions required for a laparoscopic varicocelectomy.

3 Three 10mm ports are placed according to the diagram in Chapter 8 (Fig. 8.1). The subumbilical port is used for the telescope. A 30° telescope is sometimes useful if the sigmoid colon is full, because this allows visualization over the top and down onto the testicular vessels. The two secondary ports along the lateral edges of the rectus sheath are for manipulative and dissecting instruments. The use of two 10mm ports allows the clip applier to be introduced through either of them. The ports should be fixed with either grips or purse-string sutures.

4 The operator stands on the contralateral side of the patient whilst the camera-holder stands on the ipsilateral side.

5 The monitors should be at the bottom corners of the operating table.

6 Adhesions to the sigmoid colon may need to be divided on the left-hand side before the testicular vessels become evident. The vas should be easily identified leaving the internal inguinal ring and coursing medially and downwards. The site of spermatic vessel dissection must be well away from the vas. The peritoneum is picked up and incised longitudinally for 2 cm just lateral to the testicular vessels. A 1 cm incision perpendicular to this in the peritoneum over the vessels allows greater exposure (Fig. 9.1). The internal spermatic fascia then requires a separate longitudinal incision before the individual veins can be identified. Close attention is required to discriminate between veins and the fine accompanying lymphatics. A single or double artery will lie very close to one or two of the veins respectively, and dissection between them must be very careful. Care must be taken not to place too much tension on these vessels so that a testicular artery does not go into spasm and remains identifiable by virtue of its pulsation. The use of a laparoscopic doppler probe to identify the artery is an advantage. As each vein is identified, it should be divided between double small clips on each side. Watch the tips of the clip to prevent catching adjacent lymphatics or small nerves. Division of each vein in turn will allow closer inspection and more accurate dissection of the remaining contents of the internal spermatic fascia. Indiscriminate use of diathermy should be avoided to prevent inappropriate vessel ablation. A swab is preferable to irrigation and suction in these cases. The gauze swab should be connected to a nylon or silk retention suture via one of the ports. When all of the testicular veins have been divided, one's attention should turn to the vas. A small peritoneal incision is made over the vas and any possible dilated vasal vein obliterated with diathermy or a clip. Any possible external spermatic vein can only be seen if the peritoneum is incised directly behind the inguinal canal (Fig. 9.2). If such a vessel is present, it will arise from the medial aspects of the canal and so a small incision of just 1 cm in length at the medial end of the canal is sufficient to identify such a vein. If found, this can again be divided between clips.

Excellent haemostasis should be the norm. Any loose swabs should be withdrawn. If a bilateral varicocelectomy is required, the same ports can be used but we suggest that the operator and cameraman switch positions.

8 The ports must be removed under direct vision. All carbon dioxide is evacuated.

9 Wounds require a deep fascial suture to prevent wound-herniation. The skin can be either sutured with a subcuticular absorbable suture or steristrip. Patients require two to three hours to recover and can then be discharged home.

Complications

The laparoscopic varicocelectomy can be carried out as a day-case procedure. Only two of the patients in King's College Hospital have required an overnight stay and in both cases, this was for persistent nausea because of the use of inappropriate opiate analgesia peroperatively. Complications can otherwise be described as general to laparoscopy or specific to this procedure.

General complications

Veress needle or trocar injuries are extremely rare, probably due to the universal use of disposable equipment with safety shields. However, there are occasional reports of significant visceral and vascular injuries due to incorrect placement of the first port.

Perforation of the bifurcation of the aorta or iliac vessels is a very real but rare complication (less than 0.5%) and serves to remind us that the laparoscopic varicocelectomy must be shown to be a superior operation to its open counterparts which never carry such a catastrophic risk. Carbon dioxide absorption is not a problem because the procedure is usually over within 30–40 minutes.

In our series of 48 patients at King's College Hospital, there have been three cases of preperitoneal Veress needle malplacement and

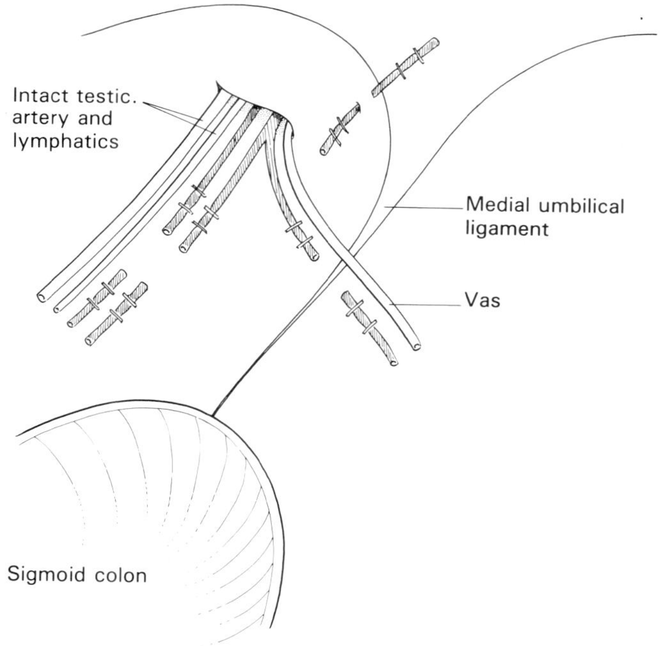

Fig. 9.2 The internal spermatic veins, sparing the lymphatics and the artery, together with the vasal and external spermatic veins, have been clipped and divided. Division is necessary to prevent recanalization. The veins rarely seem dilated in the head-down position. Inadvertent division of the testicular artery sometimes occurs, but this does not seem to have any serious clinical sequelae.

two superficial epigastric arterial incidents with the placement of secondary ports. Neither of these two types of complication have prevented a successful completion of the procedure and all occurred in the hands of relatively inexperienced staff.

Malpositioning of the Veress needle into the preperitoneal space can still sometimes produce a false-negative infusion and aspiration test. One should be alerted to this problem when the initial insufflation pressure rises immediately to 12 mm of mercury or above. Early identification of this complication will allow the Veress needle to be placed into the peritoneum or, if necessary, at a distant site. The slow recognition of this complication leads to preperitoneal insufflation and it is thereafter more difficult to insert any of the ports and the patient is often uncomfortable postoperatively with superficial emphysema.

A superficial inferior epigastric artery rupture is usually only noticed upon removal of a port because the cannula has been tamponading the damaged artery. A clue to its damage sometimes comes from blood slowly trickling down the cannula inside the patient. If this is the case, a suture should be placed through the whole abdominal wall around the suspected site. This is best achieved by using a Stamey needle under direct intraperitoneal visualization. The suture can be threaded into the eye of the needle after two passes and the two ends brought onto the outside of the abdominal wall and tied. Quite large haematomas can form in the rectus sheath if this complication fails to be noticed, sometimes producing a drop in haemoglobin of 1–2 g/dl.

Specific complications

There have been no specific complications in our series of patients at King's College Hospital. Aaberg *et al.* (1991), Hagood *et al.* (1992) and Donovan & Winfield (1992a, 1992b) have all reported a series where there is an absence of specific complications relating to the varicocelectomy, which reflects the ease of the technique and its safety once the ports have been inserted.

Donovan has felt that the risk, although small, of trocar injury has led him to utilize the open Hasson technique for the introduction of the first telescope port.

Discussion of results

Both Hagood *et al.* (1992) and Donovan & Winfield (1992a) have published results of their experience with the laparoscopic varicocelectomy. Hagood's series includes 10 patients with a mixture of clinical indications for a varicocelectomy. Four of these patients had bilateral varicocelectomies. There was no residual or recurrent varicocele demonstrated on either clinical or doppler examination in this series and complications were minimal. His technique was to identify the veins in as accurate a way as possible, and he was able to identify and leave the testicular artery preserved in each case. The procedure was particularly valuable for those patients with bilateral varicoceles because the same ports could be used. Donovan's series contained 14 patients. Five were bilateral. The clinical indications were all for oligospermia. Again, there were no recurrences in this series on follow-up, but this was based on clinical examination only. A return to normal activity was measured and there was found to be a mean of 3.4 days after the procedure. Several of the patients had undergone previous abdominal surgery and his recommendation is to introduce the first 10mm port by the open Hasson technique. The adhesions from an appendicectomy are rarely significant unless the patient gives a history of preceding peritonitis and this is not an absolute indication for the Hasson technique but may be preferred by the very cautious.

On the other hand, a more significant predictor of intra-abdominal adhesions such as a lower midline or paramedian incision should be a contraindication to a laparoscopic varicocelectomy. There seems little point in carefully dissecting these and both prolonging a simple operation and increasing the morbidity. An alternative open-groin approach would on balance be best in these cases.

One can, however, follow the logic of Donovan's later argument (Donovan & Winfield 1992b) where he recommends that all pelvic laparoscopy be initiated with the open introduction of the first port to avoid absolutely the rare vascular injuries caused sometimes by the

Veress needle, more often by the blind introduction of the first port a shielded trocar is not used. This debate will have to continue until the 'safety' ports have been evaluated over many years.

Donovan & Winfield (1992b) have also gone on to compare the use of the Nd:YAG laser for dissection and coagulation and have found this to be superior to using scissors and diathermy but if this is a rerun of the laparoscopic cholecystectomy–laser study then the minimal benefits will be overridden by the extra costs and frustration of wearing protective eyewear.

In our own series at King's College Hospital, we have seen the evolution of a new procedure that reflects the advantages that a laparoscopic technique brings. Our first 15 patients underwent mass ligation of the spermatic veins. The testicular artery was not identified in six cases although there were no unwanted sequelae of testicular pain or subsequent atrophy. The second series of 15 patients underwent a slightly more sophisticated laparoscopic procedure where the veins were identified, clipped and divided behind the retroperitoneum, the peritoneum was opened behind the inguinal canal and any external spermatic vein (three cases) if present was also clipped and any dilated vasal veins were also similarly dealt with (two cases). This was, to all intents and purposes, a much more complete and radical ablation of the venous drainage of the testicle. In this group of patients, there were no recurrences on either clinical or doppler follow-up after six months which is in contrast to four recurrent varicoceles in our first series (27%). The disadvantage of the more complete venous ablation was the formation of lymphatic hydroceles in three cases (20%).

In order to avoid this complication and yet still achieve the same high standard of success for the varicocelectomy, we have concentrated on using the laparoscope as an endoscopic operating microscope. In our most recent series of 10 cases, the same degree of venous ablation has been achieved but at the same time, the cord has been much more carefully dissected with finer instruments and small clips have been used. The testicular artery and associated lymphatics have all been identified and left intact. This has produced the ideal result of complete success in eradicating the varicocele and we have also avoided the complication of a lymphatic hydrocele. This seems to be a good example of how a laparoscopic procedure should not merely be a copy of a previously described open counterpart. However, we will not see the additional benefits of using the laparoscope as an endoscopic operating microscope until the telescopes themselves have further increased magnification and the instrumentation becomes more refined for delicate dissection. The length of the operation in all surgeons' hands has become dramatically shorter with experience, and no more than 30–40 minutes should be needed for a unilateral varicocelectomy.

The advantage as stated above of a bilateral varicocelectomy carried out through the same ports means that this only adds a mere 10–15 minutes on to the procedure if this is indicated. The cost of using disposable equipment throughout the procedure has been criticized in the past, and where we have to compete in terms of health economics with other simple day-case alternatives, the use only of a nondisposable first telescope port and disposable sharp microscissors seems indicated now.

The future of the laparoscopic varicocelectomy is much more secure because it has now evolved into a refined technique that matches the gold standard set by Goldstein *et al.* (1992) but at the same time reduces the trauma of access and so allows the patient to return to normal activities much quicker than even the most minor open alternative.

References

Aaberg R.A., Vancaille T.G., Schuessler W.W. (1991) Laparoscopic varicocele ligation: A new technique. *Fertility and Sterility*, **56**, 776.

Ahlberg N.E., Bartley O., Chidekel N. (1966) Right and left gonadal veins: An anatomical and statistical study. *Acta Radiologica*, **4**, 593.

Beck E.M., Schlegel P.N., Goldstein M. (1992) Intraoperative varicocele anatomy: A macroscopic and microscopic study. *Journal of Urology*, **148**, 1190–4.

Belgrano E., Puppo P., Quattrini S., Trombetta C., Giuliani L. (1984) The role of venography and sclerotherapy in the management of varicocele. *European Urology*, **10**, 124.

Donovan J.F., Winfield H.N. (1992a) Laparoscopic varix ligation. *Journal of Urology*, **147**, 77.

Donovan J.F., Winfield H.N. (1992b) Laparoscopic varix ligation with the Nd:YAG laser. *Journal of Endourology*, **6**: 2, 165–71.

Goldstein M., Gilbert B., Dicker A.P., Dwosk J., Gnecco C. (1992) Microsurgical inguinal varicocoelectomy with delivery of the testis: An artery and lymphatic sparing technique. *Journal of Urology*, **148**, 1808–11.

Greenberg S.H. (1977) Varicocele and male fertility. *Fertility and Sterility*, **28**, 699.

Hagood P.G., Mehan D.J., Wrischeck J.H., Andrus C.H., Parra R.O. (1992) Laparoscopic varicocelectomy: Preliminary report of a new technique. *Journal of Urology*, **147**, 73.

Ivanissevich O. (1960) Left varicocele due to reflux: Experience with 4,470 operative cases in forty-two years: *Journal of the International College of Surgeons*, **34**, 742.

Kaufman S.L., Kadir S., Barth K.H., Smyth J.W., Walsh P.C., White R.I. Jr (1983) Mechanisms of recurrent varicocele after balloon occlusion or surgical ligation of the internal spermatic vein. *Radiology*, **147**, 435.

Murray R.R. Jr, Mitchell S.E., Kadir S. *et al.* (1986) Comparison of recurrent varicocele anatomy following surgery and percutaneous balloon occlusion. *Journal of Urology*, **135**, 286.

Palomo A. (1949) Radical cure of varicocele by a new technique: Preliminary report. *Journal of Urology*, **61**, 604.

Porst H., Bähren W., Lenz M., Altwein J.E. (1984) Percutaneous sclerotherapy of varicoceles—an alternative to conventional surgical methods. *British Journal of Urology*, **56**, 73.

Rothman C.M., Newmark H. III, Karson R.A. (1981) The recurrent varicocele—a poorly recognised problem. *Fertility and Sterility*, **35**, 552.

Sayfan J., Adam Y.G., Soffer Y. (1981) A natural 'venous bypass' causing post-operative recurrence of a varicocele. *Journal of Andrology*, **2**, 108.

Szabo R., Kessler R. (1984) Hydrocoele following internal spermatic vein ligation: A retrospective study and review of the literature. *Journal of Urology*, **132**, 924.

10: Laparoscopic Herniorraphy

M.J. COPTCOAT AND A.D. JOYCE

Introduction

Transabdominal repair of an inguinal hernia is not a new concept and many surgeons will readily perform such a procedure if associated with a concomitant laparotomy (La Roque 1932, Ger 1982, Marcy 1987). The laparoscopic approach to hernia repair is a natural progression from this concept. It has the advantage of avoiding a muscle-cutting incision and so postoperative pain is minimal. A tension-free prosthesis is fixed to the preperitoneal surface with metal clips to accomplish closure of the internal inguinal ring and to strengthen the weak posterior inguinal wall. This is similar to the open technique described by Nyhus *et al.* (1988). This laparoscopic placement could conceivably be the same for direct, indirect or even femoral hernias. There are very few large series of laparoscopic hernia repairs and certainly no long-term results are available as yet, but short-term results are very encouraging (Popp 1990).

The technique involves incising the peritoneum medially and laterally from the internal ring with point diathermy or scissors around the medial edge of the internal ring. The sac is then dissected free and either left open or closed (Ger *et al.* 1990) with an endoloop. A mesh plug can be introduced into the indirect hernial defect or a posterior wall herniorrhaphy can be undertaken by stapling a second mesh.

Laparoscopic instrumentation

1 High-flow carbon dioxide insufflator
2 CCD camera and at least one monitor
3 Veress needle (safety)
4 0° 10mm laparoscope (30° optional)
5 One 10mm port plus two 12mm ports with grips and converters/downsizers
6 Laparoscopic curved microscissors (diathermy connection)
7 Laparoscopic soft grasping forceps
8 Laparoscopic curved dissecting forceps
9 Laparoscopic hernia stapler
10 Nonabsorbable polypropylene mesh

Technique

1 Under a general anaesthetic with muscle paralysis and assisted

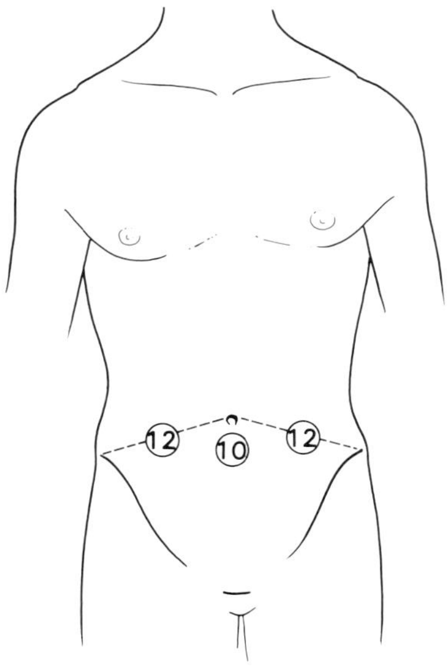

Fig. 10.1 Sites of the 10mm telescope port and two 12mm ports for manipulative and dissecting instruments in a laparoscopic inguinal herniorraphy.

ventilation, the patient is put in a supine position with a 20–25° head-down tilt (Fig. 4.1a). A catheter is not usually required if the patient's bladder has recently emptied. Hip flexion is not required.

2 Formation of the pneumoperitoneum (Fig. 4.1): the Veress needle is inserted at an angle of 45° into the empty pelvis. The position should be checked for aspiration by infusion of 5ml of saline and the intra-abdominal pressure should remain below 12ml of mercury during insufflation. In the hands of inexperienced laparoscopists, the disposable Veress needles with a safety shield are safer. Previous major abdominal surgery is a relative contraindication. A previous appendicectomy is unlikely to have produced difficult intra-abdominal adhesions, but anything more significant than this may produce an unnecessarily difficult procedure out of proportion to the open alternatives for a herniorrhaphy.

3 A 10mm port for the telescope is placed just below the umbilicus. Two 12mm ports are inserted along the lateral edges of the rectus sheath and these are for manipulative and dissecting instruments (Fig. 10.1). The use of two 12mm ports allows the sta,pling device to be inserted from either side which sometimes facilitates easier access to certain parts of the herniorrhaphy. The ports should be fixed either with grips or purse-string sutures.

4 The operator stands on the contralateral side of the patient whilst the camera holder stands on the ipsilateral side (Fig. 8.1).

5 The monitors should be at the bottom corners of the operating table.

6 Adhesions to the sigmoid colon may need to be divided on the left-hand side. An indirect hernial sac should be circumcised at the internal inguinal ring after the contents have been withdrawn back into the abdomen. The terminal portion is left free.

7 The peritoneum is then incised behind the back wall of the inguinal canal with scissors. The inferior epigastric vessels sometimes require division between clips if it looks as if they will prevent precise placement of the mesh. The peritoneum is dissected to reveal

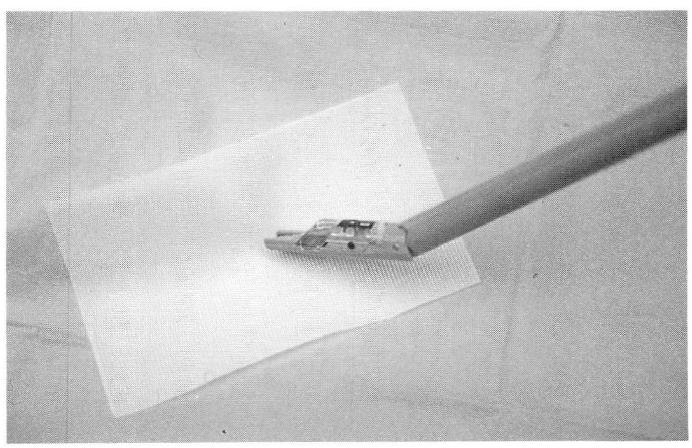

Fig. 10.2 A herniorraphy stapler that can be angled to produce a better contact.

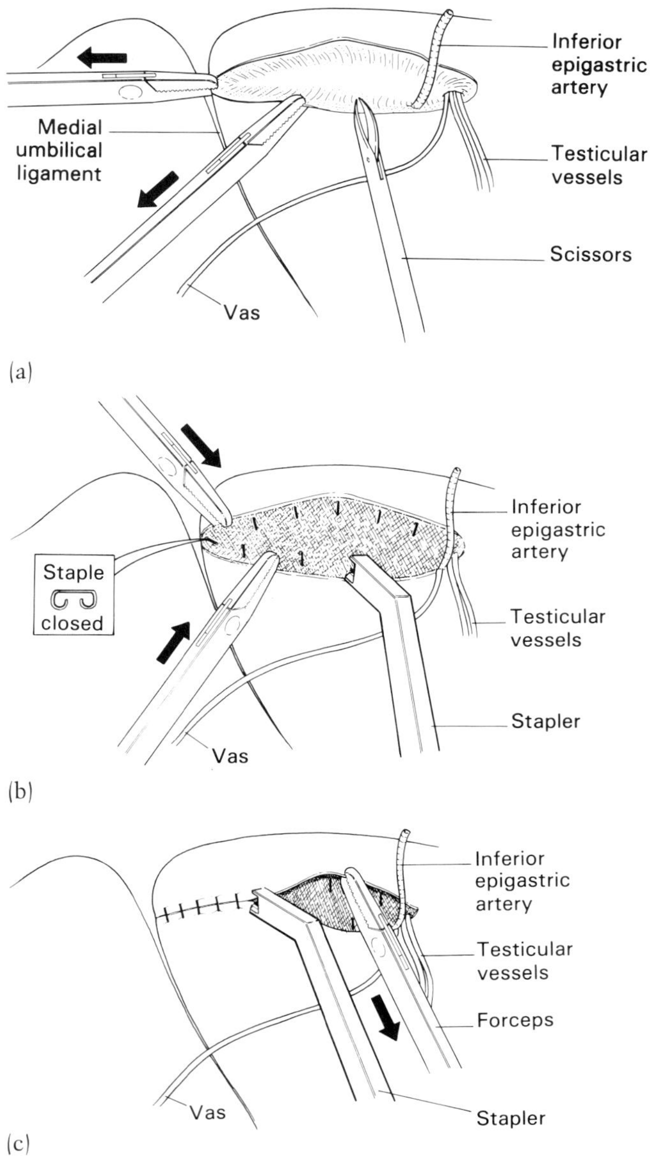

Fig. 10.3 (a) The peritoneum is dissected to reveal enough space for a mesh plug behind the weak posterior wall of the inguinal canal. (b) The tailored piece of mesh is stapled to the inguinal ligament below the conjoint tendon. (c) The peritoneum is brought back and stapled to cover the mesh.

enough space for the mesh (Fig. 10.3a). An approximate template can be measured using the known length of the forceps or scissors. The required size of mesh is then inserted and placed up against the back wall of the inguinal canal. It is stapled to the inguinal ligament below, the pubic tubercle medially and internal oblique aponeurosis superiorly (Fig. 10.3b). The stapler can be angulated to fire the staples perpendicular to the structures and if this is not possible, introduction of the stapler through the opposite side usually helps. The peritoneum is then brought back over to cover the mesh and can be either closed with a continuous suture or with further staples (Fig. 10.3c). The latter is much simpler and quicker. A direct hernia does not obviously require any dissection of a sac and the defect in the posterior wall of the inguinal canal can be enhanced by asking an assistant to place two or three fingers externally into the defect and dissection can take place around them. Otherwise the technique for herniorrhaphy is indentical to that of an indirect hernia.

8 The ports must be removed under direct vision. All carbon dioxide is evacuated.

9 All wounds require a deep fascial suture to prevent wound-hernias. The skin can be either sutured with a subcuticular absorbable suture or steristrip. Patients require two or three hours to recover and can then be discharged home. Patients should refrain from lifting more than a briefcase for three weeks.

Discussion

There is no doubt that currently available stapling instrumentation makes the laparoscopic herniorrhaphy a simple and straightforward procedure. However, its long-term results are unknown but earlier results are very encouraging and point to a recurrence rate that is at least as low as with an open herniorrhaphy (Corbitt 1991, Nolen *et al.* 1992). Unfortunately, the present stapling devices are quite expensive and it is difficult to rationalize this procedure against a day-case open herniorrhaphy, especially when done under local anaesthesia.

When a laparoscopic alternative drastically changes the morbidity and hospital stay, the increase in operating time and equipment is irrelevant, but in the case of a herniorrhaphy, this contrast is not apparent. The patients definitely experience far less postoperative discomfort following a laparoscopic herniorrhaphy and this is enough to keep most of us open-minded. The answer probably lies in nondisposable instrumentation being developed that will reduce the operating costs.

Discussion still takes place regarding the indirect sac and many surgeons are beginning to leave the sac free after excision and pack the inguinal canal with a Marlex mesh folded into a fan configuration. This is becoming the method of choice for treating indirect hernias whilst the stapling of a simple mesh over the posterior wall will probably be the best solution for direct inguinal hernias. Further follow-up is required to confirm these speculative thoughts.

References

Corbitt, J.D. (1991) Laparoscopic herniorrhaphy. *Surgical Laparoscopy and Endoscopy*, **1**, 23–25.

Ger R. (1982) The management of certain abdominal hernias by intra-abdominal closure of the neck. *Annals of the Royal College of Surgeons of England*, **64**, 342–4.

Ger R, Monroe K, Duvivier R *et al*: (1990) Management of indirect inguinal hernias by laparoscopic closure of the neck of the sac. *American Journal of Surgery*, **159**, 370–2.

LaRoque G.P. (1932) The intra-abdominal method of removing inguinal and femoral herniae. *Archives of Surgery*, **24**, 189–203.

Marcy H.O. (1987) The cure of hernia. *Journal of the American Medical Association*, **8**, 589–92.

Nolen M., Melichar R., Jennings W.C., McGee J. (1992) Use of a Marlex fan in the repair of direct and indirect hernias by laparoscopy. *Journal of Laparoendoscopic Surgery*, **2**, (2), 1061–4.

Nyhus L.M., Pollak R., Bombeck T.C., Conahue P.E. (1988) The preperitoneal approach and prosthetic buttress repair for recurrent hernia. *Annals of Surgery*, **208**, 733–7.

Popp L.W. (1990) Endoscopic patch repair of inguinal hernia in a female patient. *Surgical Endoscopy*, **4**, 10-12.

Index

Page numbers in **bold** refer to tables, those in *italic* to figures.